ENDORSEMENTS

"Knowing Mark for more than a decade, I have witnessed many of the struggles and the victories that led him to write this book. In *UNDRESSED*, he writes from a place of unhindered honesty, sharing his journey through the difficulties of reality television and weight loss, and ultimately shedding the person he used to be to become the person he was meant to be. This book will give perspective, encouragement, and most importantly, hope for your journey."

— **Michael Mills**: Connections Pastor at Inland Church, Spokane, WA

"Even though millions of fans of The Biggest Loser know Mark from his epic role in an epic season of the show, the "back story" of Mark's journey overshadows anything that happened in front of the camera. The story-behind-the-story is about a God who relentlessly pursues us, and will use anything—including a weight-loss reality show—to strip away the lies we live by, creating a hunger for Him instead. And then He offers Himself, and His truths, to fill that void. Read Mark's story, and you'll find what you've always been looking for."

— **Rick Lawrence**: Editor of GROUP Magazine and author of Sifted and Shrewd, Loveland, CO

"Mark does an outstanding job of bringing us into his story so we can better understand what it means to live outside of ourselves – pursuing the heart of God."

> — **Matt Storer**: President and CEO of VisionTrust International, Chairman of Christian Alliance for Orphans and Food for Orphans, Colorado Springs, CO

"Mark Cornelison has penned a powerful tale of his "Biggest Loser" journey and what he learned by being forced out of his comfort zone. There are lessons here for all of us. The most important one? That God is in charge of our journey, and He knows best. Despite the initial fears and concerns Mark had, he emerged a big winner in all the ways that truly matter."

> — **Dennis Welch**, CEO of Articulāte, and author of "So…what are you saying?" Austin, TX

"This is a powerful story of challenge, courage, growth, and victory intertwined with the greatest story of all time…God's love and redemption of humanity. After reading this book you will feel empowered to make changes in your life and you will also be reminded of God's love, mercy, and purpose that is uniquely yours. Mark will have you laughing and crying at his Biggest Loser adventure while encouraging your heart with truth from Scripture. If you need to be reminded that there is hope in your struggle and that the Creator of the universe loves you just as you are, this book is for you!"

> — **Robin Renfrew**: Professor at Lubbock Christian University, Lubbock, TX

"Mark's story is not just about losing weight. It's about shedding the baggage of destructive thinking that weighs us down. And it's about living in God's grace and letting it transform us from the inside out. I've watched this message radically change Mark's life, his family and those around him. Mark is the real deal - listen to what he has to say."

— **Dr. Bill Yarger**: retired pastor and seminary vice-president, Phoenix, AZ

"Mark Cornelison's insights in this book are nothing short of genius! Mark's account of his own personal journey engages the reader in an authentic and vulnerable way! This is the first book about a person's weight loss story that doesn't attempt to offer a "band-aid" solution to the problem. Instead, Mark addresses the root of the problem. Actually, this book addresses the root of most, if not all, problems. Those who embrace the truths that are presented in this book will walk away transformed."

— **Allen "Buddy" Shuh**: Connections Pastor at The Journey Community Church, Wayne, MI

"One of the most freeing things to do in life is to replace the lies we tell ourselves with the truth that comes from God's Word. Mark captures this freedom in this refreshing, raw, and authentic book. This book encourages the Church to be living proof that God matters and people matter. And when we live out this truth, we can impact people with Mark's own words, "Do what you need to do today to be the person you are meant to be tomorrow."

— **J. Chad Barrett**, Director of Child Evangelism Fellowship, Houston, TX, and founder of IEWorks, LLC.

Endorsements

"Mark does an excellent job of taking his audaciously public moments and boiling them down to gentle, private truths for the reader. His private journey sparked a public passion for people. During a wrinkle in his personal timeline that could have been solely self-focused, God drew a vastly grand masterpiece that focused on people and changed Mark's life forever. He may have lost the weight, but he gained so much more…and in the generous, affable way that Mark has – he shares it with each of us in this great book!

> — **Darren Sutton**: youth pastor, author of Everyone's Called to Youth Ministry, and fellow fat guy, Corpus Christi, TX

"I have shared 10 years of friendship and ministry with Mark Cornelison, and I heard his excuses many times about losing weight. Seemingly out of the blue an opportunity to be a part of The Biggest Loser became a reality, and the real Mark was UNDRESSED before the world and redressed not only physically, but also spiritually. Read this honest, loving, and beautiful story that "undresses" our search for what matters most in this life."

> — **Tray Morgan**: Associate Pastor, Redemption Anglican Church, Frisco, TX

"No one likes to be exposed, literally put on display for all to see…especially in front of a large audience. I would often joke with Mark about how terrifying that must have been on The Biggest Loser. However, exposure is what all of us need as we struggle toward the authentic life that Christ desires for us. I am thrilled that Mark has given us UNDRESSED to remind us that when we look in the life's mirror and often don't like what we see, we must remember what God sees and what he desires for our life. This book reminds me of the truths of Hebrews 12:1-2 and I encourage you to remember the same as you run with endurance the race marked out for you."

— **J. Roger Davis**: President of Student Life,
Birmingham, AL

"Being uncomfortable is not something that any of us choose. But it's exactly what most of us need. In *UNDRESSED*, Mark lets us walk along as God takes him to a place where he is uncomfortable physically, emotionally, and spiritually. And Mark shares practical, simple, biblical insights to help us begin that journey as well. If you have ever struggled with purpose or identity, this book is a must read."

— **Tracy Ward**: Pastor of Youth & Missions,
Kingfisher, OK

"It is rare in the world that we live in to find someone doing something without ulterior motives. We not only expect it, we look for it. Mark writes this book out of a selfless desire to use his experiences and knowledge to share tools that will help bring healing, health, and deeper, richer relationships to others. This book is as authentic as Mark himself."

— **Deb Juliot**, Actress, Community Leader,
Omaha, NE

UNDRESSED

Taking Everything Off and Putting on What Matters Most

BY

MARK CORNELISON

LUCIDBOOKS

UNDRESSED - Taking Everything Off and Putting on What Matters Most

Arrangement copyrighted © Mark Cornelison

Published by Lucid Books in Brenham, TX.
www.LucidBooks.net

First Printing: 2014

ISBN-10: 1935909924
ISBN-13: 978-1-935909-92-7

Special Sales: Most Lucid Books titles are available in special quantity discounts. Custom imprinting or excerpting can also be done to fit special needs. Contact Lucid Books at info@lucidbooks.net.

DEDICATION

Dedicated to the most patient, supportive, and motivating woman in the world, Cathy. Thank you for being my best friend and loving wife. I love you and thank God for sending us on this most excellent adventure together.

TABLE OF CONTENTS

Table of Contents

ACKNOWLEDGMENTS

The fact that I have actually written a book is a miraculous thing. However, once you read it you will realize this took lots of people to make it happen. I do not really know how many people really read the acknowledgments, but it doesn't matter. I just cannot put this out there and leave the image that somehow I did this by myself, so here goes:

First and foremost, I thank God for the life and experiences I have had that brought me to this point. This book is not about me. It is about the work of a gracious and loving God who not only gave me the gift of His Son, Jesus, but who also gives that gift to anyone who asks. This book is His, and I pray that it is used to help encourage the people He created, as well as point them solely to Him.

I definitely have to thank my family. My amazing wife, Cathy, my daughter and my youngest son, who willingly gave me up for 6 months on this journey. Once that part ended, a whole new world opened up and still they have lovingly allowed us all to be thrown into an incredibly visible public life. Thank you guys for believing in me and making this ride so fun. I love each of you more than you could ever imagine.

Of course I cannot leave out my oldest son, Chism. We have shared an experience like few fathers and sons have.

Acknowledgments

You put yourself out there with me even though we could not have imagined what this road would look like. You were and continue to be one of my greatest encouragers and motivators as the journey continues. I love you, Chiz! I will always be proud and thankful for taking this crazy ride with you.

Included in my appreciation is all the rest of my family: an incredibly supportive mom, dad, a great sister, wonderful in-laws (including sisters-in-law & brothers-in-law), nieces, and nephews. Thank you guys for loving me through this and beyond.

A great amount of appreciation goes out to everyone associated with The Biggest Loser, you guys have given me my life back and I will forever be grateful. From Holland Weathers and Kerry Shanahan who saw something in us in that casting call in Austin, TX, to all the fantastic people in front and behind the camera. Dolvett, Tracy (the rockstar), Allison, Cardio Chris, Bob, Sandy, Rachel, Chrissy, Joel, Mallory, Catherine, Lane, Caitlin, Justin, Crabby, Alexis, Kat, Joel R., Curtis, Jorie, Nolte, Mario, DAVE!, A-Ro, Kristen, Ryan, Dr. H, Todd, and all the fantastic story producers; thank you for laughing, loving, and putting up with me during this phenomenal change of life. You are each part of this story. This obviously also includes my fellow contestants, thank you guys for the ups and downs. Those days revealed something about all of us and continue to shape who we are. I'm proud to have started the journey with every one of you.

Thank you as well to all the staff and friends at Faith Bible Church who took a chance in letting their youth pastor disappear for half a year. You showed that grace is not just a message you teach; it is part of the DNA of your church body.

I want to give credit as well to all my friends who have been so encouraging through this time. Whether you are a

Acknowledgments

new friend or an old one, I am thankful for your continued outreach to my family and me.

Mega shout out to all my youth worker connections across this country. I pray I represented us well! Group Mag, IT3ers, and Simply Healthy peeps keep the faith and don't settle for mediocrity. Our Savior and our students need people like us to challenge them as they walk towards the Kingdom.

If you feel forgotten then know I am thankful for you too. Blame it on my age or something…

EDITORIAL ACKNOWLEDGEMENT

One thing I've learned from writing this book is that there are definitely some things I can't do by myself. Early on, I thought I could just make this thing happen without much help but then I realized how big the task was before me.

As I prayed through the process, I was led to a fantastic publisher who then introduced me to Carol Jones who would come alongside as my editor. There is no question that her involvement and expertise has made all the difference.

I've appreciated the ease of communication and the honesty I have received while working with Carol. She has been instrumental in guiding the flow of this project as well sharing valuable and professional advice.

When my next book comes along I don't even have to hesitate when I say whom the editor will be. Thanks, Carol. Looking forward to what the next project will be!

Contact information for Ms. Jones
Carol Jones
Benchmark Creative Resources.com
Carol@WeSetTheMark.com
770-362-6000

FOREWORD

"My goal in life, be better than yesterday,
and continue to change lives one Rep at a time."

"When I first met Mark and his son, Chism, on set at the "Ranch" for season 13 of The Biggest Loser, I instantly gravitated towards him. He had a quiet and confident disposition, and a love for his son I could relate to.

More importantly he had a look in eyes that simply said, "I'm ready." Ready to take life back, ready to be healthy, ready to forgive and forget, ready to start all over!

I saw God in him, and I still do to this day. Since his time on the Ranch, Mark and I have talked, we've prayed, and he has found the balance between, physical, mental, and spiritual health.

Mark's perspective is extremely genuine! If you're looking to be inspired, motivated, or pushed, follow his story and you'll know what I learned from the moment we met."

— **Dolvett Quince**,
Trainer for NBC's The Biggest Loser,
Los Angeles, CA

PREFACE

If you are looking for a fitness and weight-loss book this is not it. Now I fully believe that the principles outlined here can help one lose weight and get healthy, but these have much deeper and far-reaching eternal implications.

What you can lose and gain here will make a greater impact on your life than just changing how you look from the outside. There is so much more to you than your appearance, so real life change cannot come without looking at the physical, mental, emotional, and spiritual sides of who you really are.

God is really big. This is not just something church people are supposed to say, He is really big. Not just the token way we hear people say that they serve a "big" God. Big in the sense that He has a unique plan and purpose for every person on this planet. There is no need for us to try to imitate His plan and purpose in someone else's life because He is big enough to have a specific journey for each of us. Our stories should not be something that others want to duplicate; rather they should inspire others to seek out God's individual plan for themselves.

So this is my story. A true story of an experience that has profoundly changed my life, but not just in the way you may expect. This story is greater than what happened during a reality television show. It is a message of grace, truth, and conviction, and about how we should view the world around us. My hope is not that you try and copy my journey, but that you will step forward towards our big God to seek out your own journey.

Maybe your issue is your weight, but maybe not. What lies ahead is truth that has the ability to overcome any obstacle. This is a new day, a new beginning, and the first step on a road with many challenges but many more rewards.

So let's get started.

INTRODUCTION

"No man can put on the robes of Christ's righteousness till he has taken off his own."

– C.H. Spurgeon

Sometimes it is so easy to look at someone else's life, someone else's story, and think, "Man, they have a great story to tell. I wish I had a story like that, a purpose in life as amazing as theirs certainly seems to be." I know those thoughts all too well, because like most people, I've had them.

For me, my story is fairly simple. Growing up in a great home with an amazing family pretty well describes my life. We were a family that loved Jesus, loved others, and tried our best to live out our faith in a way that pleased God. Like most kids from the Bible belt, I was at the church anytime the doors were open, and not because I was forced to be there. I enjoyed it.

Later in life, I married an amazing woman and had three awesome kids, all while spending 17+ years in a ministry that I loved. I wouldn't say our life was idyllic (no one's is). We've definitely had our issues along the way, but I can honestly say that I have not had a rough life, *at all*.

Yet, despite all of the goodness in my life, I had this thought in the back of my mind that there had to be greater things on the horizon for me. As good as my life was, I felt somehow unfulfilled. For a long time, I ignored those feelings and reminded myself I had a pretty good life. Trust me, in my years of ministry, I'd *seen* some people with rough lives, people who *needed* to look out on the horizon for a better life, but that wasn't me. I was doing okay as far life went.

So why was this feeling there? If my life was so good, then why did I always have this sense that I was made for more? Sometimes when I heard people tell amazing stories of how they'd been freed from some terrible addiction or survived some hardship in life, I'd find myself longing for the impact they seemed to be making.

How was I going to make an impact in the world? I didn't have some amazing story of redemption to tell. I was an ordinary guy, living a decent life in American suburbia. And although I worked really hard at convincing myself I could make a difference in my little neck of the woods, for some reason this feeling—this overwhelming sense of longing—was there, telling me God had created me for a purpose, and I was not yet living it out.

The Search Began

I began trying to figure it out.

I loved life as a youth pastor, but maybe that was where I needed to make a change. I enjoyed teaching and speaking, so maybe I was supposed to branch out and speak? Maybe my next step was to be a lead pastor or a teaching pastor? For a season, I even tried seminary, but that just did not seem to fit my passions either.

As a family we loved missions, so maybe we were supposed to move to a foreign land and live among tribes while sharing the gospel? I mean, come on, it doesn't get much more impactful than that. And yet it never seemed like the time or place was ever revealed to us.

So, I kept searching, kept trying to figure out what I was supposed to be doing with my life.

Looking back, I realize now that what I was doing was what many of us do. I was trying to create value in my life without stepping even one foot outside of the comfortable life I had created for myself. Funny thing was, I wanted so desperately to live out the calling God had in my life, but I was missing a pretty important step in the process.

The Missing Step

One of the hazards of working in ministry is that sometimes we think since "God-things" surround us all the time, then we are somehow constantly in touch with His purpose and will. We believe the lie that makes us think that we do not need to intentionally seek Him because we are working for Him. It's like 'faith-osmosis.' Basically if it surrounds me, it must be seeping into me, so I do not have to be intentional like everyone else.

I was searching for what God wanted me to do, but I wasn't asking God what *He* wanted me to do. At some point in my search, I realized that I needed to stop and give my thoughts and my search for purpose to the One who had all the answers. So one day, I simply gave it up. "If there really is something more out there, then I want You to reveal it to me. I am tired of trying to guess."

No one could have ever imagined the crazy adventure that

lay ahead. That simple prayer opened up a world that I never could have dreamed of, and this book is part of the message of what I am still learning as the journey continues.

Turns out, while I was convinced there were things that I needed to add to my life, I quickly saw that this story was to begin with me taking many things off first. I was about to be undressed in a very public and life-changing way.

PART ONE

Taking Off What's False

CHAPTER 1

What's the Point?

"I've failed over and over and over again in my life and that is why I succeed."

– Michael Jordan

*O*ur family has always been reality show fans. So for us to even consider trying out for one was not a stretch. However, thanks to a life of poor health habits, the decision about which one to try out for was an easy one. I was not exactly going to succeed at running around the world looking for clues; being abandoned on a desert island with strangers was too scary (although the weight loss plan is pretty impressive...); and I definitely was not going to live in a camera-filled house (so I thought...).

So while watching a season of our favorite weight-loss show, one of the commercials invited us to apply to be contestants. We decided to give it a try. Well, actually I decided to give it a try. (Convincing my son was going to be a whole other issue.)

To help you understand, I need to insert a little history. My oldest son, Chism, struggles with his weight just like me. However, *his situation is different. At nine years old, Chism fell off a 7-foot wall and completely shattered his right ankle. Over the next six years, he underwent seven surgeries and spent a great deal of time in a wheelchair and on crutches. Once he turned 15, the ankle was cleared and the surgeries ended. Unfortunately, his years of limited activity had taken its toll on his health. Due to years of playing video games while waiting for the next doctor's appointment, he had gained weight and also missed out on years developmentally, compared to where many of his friends were.*

Chism and I had tried to work out and lose weight many times, but either through discouragement or laziness we both gave up and ended up worse than we were before we ever started. On some level mentally, we both had about decided it was not worth the effort any longer. The minimal success was not worth the pain of going back time and time again.

So that's when this idea came... how about doing something crazy like taking our greatest struggle in life and displaying it in front of millions of people on national TV? Needless to say, Chism was not a fan. I still remember him feeling defeated and simply asking, "Dad, what's the point?"

So What IS the Point?

Have you ever asked yourself this question? I know I have, especially regarding my life. I typically ask this when I've failed at taking care of myself (it helps me justify my poor habits). The question is almost always followed by a string of unhealthy thoughts that help me rationalize giving up altogether. See if you identify with any of these...

The Defeated Thought: *What's the point? I've tried and failed. I've tried again and failed again. What's the point* *of trying once more when I'll likely just fail once more? I will just resign myself to the fact that I will never get this under control.*

The "I am Human" Thought: *What's the point? I'm human. I've got problems. Everyone battles something so this is my something. I've wanted this thing to go away for a long time, but it's still here, so I'm just going to have to learn to live with it.*

The Spiritual Thought: *What's the point? This body is just a tent, it's weak, and it's temporary. My eternal body is in heaven where I will not have to think about emotional or physical struggles.*

The Honest Thought: *What's the point? I have a problem, and I wish there was some way to get this under control, but as far as I can tell, there isn't. I'm open to the idea that there is a solution, but if I'm honest with myself, I'm just not sure there's hope for me at this point.*

So then, what's the point of trying? Why seek to be healthy physically, mentally, emotionally, or spiritually? How about this? We are not being used to the fullest extent of God's potential for us when we do not take care of ourselves.

This is what it came down to for me, physically I was limited in life because I **could** not do active things with my family and friends; mentally I was limited because I **would** not do active things with them. I no longer had an attitude that was ready and willing for whatever God wanted me to do for Him.

Imagine, a teacher who will not use books, a doctor who will not work around blood, or a policeman who will not carry a weapon. Maybe they can do their job, but they will not do it well or to their full ability. This described me: a guy called to a specific task—for me, working in the lives of people—who could not fully invest *in people* because I had physically and mentally created a barrier to them because of my health.

Discovering the Way

Here's the point: Being healthy involves more than just our physical well-being. Being healthy involves our total well-being, physically, emotionally and spiritually. It allows us to experience life to the fullest, or in my case (and maybe in yours), keeps us from living the life we were created to live. That is what this story is about. It's about discovering your way to health; physical health, emotional health, and spiritual health.

I still remember how my heart hurt for Chism. The fact that he was 18 years old and ready to give up on a major part of his life pained me. As his dad, I wanted to do something, anything to bring back his passion for life...and mine as well. It took some convincing and lots of praying, but we began the process. I really believe we both started to get excited through each step, not because of the possibilities, but because it was clear God was setting something up, and we were a part of it.

People have asked me time and time again, "How were you able to miss work?" Early on this was a concern of mine as well, so as things started lining up, I began having conversations with my church where I worked out about what it would look like for me to go. I clearly remember telling the leadership that I did not think I would be gone long. I genuinely thought I might last no more than a couple of weeks.

At one point our executive pastor said, "Let's pretend like it could be longer and go ahead and get a plan together." The thought was, just in case I was gone for an extended period of time, we should see where and how that time could get covered. If I used all my vacation time for two years and personal days, that still wouldn't cover it all. But God was already working out the details.

Our church had a policy that once a pastor had served in our church for 10 years, they would earn a two-month sabbatical (retreat, leave, study time). This is often a great time for pastors to get refreshed in hopes of being better able to serve upon their return. As a pastor at my church, I was 3 years from this time of renewing, or so it seemed...

Just before I began the conversations about leaving, the leadership of the church decided that ten years was too long to wait for a pastor to receive this time of renewal. Overwhelmingly, they decided it would come at the end of every seven years of service. This meant I was immediately due two months of leave.

When the "what if" planning began, it was agreed that my two months would begin with my leaving, if and when it happened. This was a huge confirmation to me that something was going on that I could not have set up. "If we get to go..." was being changed very quickly to "When we get to go..." in mine and Chism's vocabulary.

Then it happened. We got an email asking if we would be interested in going to a casting call in Austin. Season 13 planning had begun, and it looked like they were going with "couples" so they wanted to meet us. That's when God really got my attention in an unexpected way...Chism ended up talking me into it. My son who had asked me, "What's the point?" was now convincing me why we should go. When I saw his desire and how he had changed, I could not resist. So we got up early on a Saturday morning and made the drive that ultimately changed our lives.

UNDRESSED

Sure enough, the call we had waited for finally came...we were off to sunny California for what ended up being close to six months on a life-changing adventure. We really had no idea what was in front of us. We were discovering God's answer to our problem, and it was nothing like we could have ever imagined.

MAIN POINTS TO REMEMBER

- **You were created to do something with your life.**

  You have to be healthy, not just physically, but emotionally and physically so you can do the amazing things you were created to do with your life.

- **Your excuses are excuses, just saying . . .**

  We all make excuses for why we can't do something. Just recognize that those are excuses, even common ones, and be willing to try again.

- **Don't fear failure.**

  Like many of us who have tried over and over again and failed, the fear of failure can be paralyzing. Don't let the fear of failure paralyze you. Thomas Edison failed thousands of times before he successfully created the light bulb. Failure is inevitable. Learning from our failure is called progress. Decide for yourself today that you aren't failing; you're making progress, and keep going!

Questions for discussion or thought

1. Which of the "thoughts" connects with you most deeply? Why? Is there a thought you have that isn't listed? What is it?

2. What area of your life needs the most work right now? Where do you most want to get healthy?

3. If you could become fully healthy (mentally, physically, emotionally, and spiritually) what would you like to do?

4. What passion do you have that is not being realized because of unhealthiness in your life?

CHAPTER 2

Addressing What Needs to be Undressed

"Our greatest weakness lies in giving up. The most certain way to succeed is always to try just one more time."

– Thomas A. Edison

The nervous energy was pretty thick. We had gotten the call, and now Chism and I found ourselves sitting in sunny California, in a fairly large hotel conference room surrounded by many other people whom we did not know. We all smiled nicely to one another but no one said a word, partly because we were nervous, but mostly because we weren't allowed to. We had spent the better part of two weeks being whisked around from place to place, riding silently in vans, going through all types of tests without a word to those around us.

It made sense, really; the idea was that if we made it onto the show then our first interactions together needed to be fresh, real, and honest...so we could not talk, at all. We would all be living together, so they did not want us to connect until it could all be captured for the viewing audience. So as I sat, waiting anxiously, I began to size up (no pun intended) the competition.

In one corner, we had what looked like some brothers, in another, a couple of mother/daughters, in another a couple that looked to be straight from the North Pole. This looked good for Chism and me; no other father/sons were in this group. However, I was the smallest guy there, which meant this room might have been for those who were about to head home.

Finally, in walked a team of professional looking people. They visited, they stared, then visited some more...and stared some more, until finally one of them came to the front of the room and got everyone's attention. This was the moment of truth. In a few minutes we would find out if our life was about to change drastically, or if we would politely be sent home, having made it so close to the life-altering help we all so desperately needed.

How Did I Get Here?

How in the world had I reached a place in my life where I *needed* to be sitting in that room? I mean, I was a happy guy (sort of . . . you know, minus the whole "trying to find myself" thing). I had a great relationship with my wife, my kids, and my coworkers. But I had a problem. Something, somewhere along the way had gone wrong, and here I was, sitting in this room with my son and a bunch of strangers, feeling like the next sentences spoken would either bring celebration or devastation (and either would be life-altering). How had I gotten to this place?

I'm guessing that you're thinking, "Hey Mark, that doesn't seem like such a difficult question. Your problem seems pretty obvious." And of course, I'd have to agree with you. Some people have the luxury of keeping their problems hidden from the outside world. Not so much with my problem. It was "out there" for the world to see and it was about to become even more "out there."

So how did I get to the place where I was sitting in that room?

Like you said, the answer seems simple. I was fat... overweight... obese... chunky... whatever you call it, that was me. In September of 2011, at 43 years old, I was right at 300 pounds, not a healthy weight for a guy who is just shy of 6-feet tall with a history of heart disease in his family.

But as obvious as it might seem, my weight wasn't my problem, it was just a symptom of my real problem. And on the day I sat in that sunny California hotel room, I didn't yet understand what my **real** problem was. By that time, I had given myself all kinds of excuses for why I was overweight.

- **I loved food**

  I was a guy that loved food! (Still am) I liked certain tastes and textures. I enjoyed how food made me feel. Much of my life revolved around the next meal. Looking back, I can see that food had taken an improper level of control in my life, control that I had willingly given it. Can you identify? Eating one meal, while talking about a previous meal, thinking about where you'll have the next meal? Food owned me.

- **I was getting older**

  I'd been working with students for nearly two

decades, teaching school and working in Student Ministry. I loved what I was doing, but every year seemed to get physically harder. Every year I had less energy, and they had more. I was getting older, the students were getting younger, and I couldn't be expected to keep up.

- **It was okay for me to be unhealthy**

  Unfortunately, I had bought into the stereotype that comes with life in your 40's. You know, life gets busy; job demands, family demands, lots of eating on the go, no time for yourself. I didn't feel as great as I used to, but hey, I was over 40. It was okay for me to be unhealthy because that's the way I perceived most people at my stage of life.

- **I gave to so many, I could give a little something to myself**

  Life was demanding. I'm a husband with an amazing wife who deserves my time. I work in ministry sharing in the life of many others. Add to this that as a parent of a junior high son, a high school daughter, and a college-aged son, I was on the clock 24/7. My mind had (has) a selfish side, which says, "If I am giving to others all the time then I should be able to give myself something as well." For me, that something was food. The more I served and gave to others, the more I felt I deserved to give myself something too…in the wrong way.

- **Everyone struggles with something**

  Paul (of the Bible) talks of his "thorn in the flesh" (2 Corinthians 12). For me, my weight issue was my thorn. I'd never gotten it under control and just assumed I never would. It was the thing I would always struggle with, so why try to do anything about it? Being overweight was just "my thing" and everyone has something they struggle with, right? I accepted this about myself, and for a long time told myself I was "okay" as a fat man.

Addressing What Needs to Be Undressed

It's not like I was completely unaware that I had a problem. That's why people make excuses, after all, because they KNOW they have a problem, and they need to tell themselves they are okay with it. I'd tried to make this change many times before. There had been random periods of time where I had exercised more or dieted more, lost weight (then gained weight), gotten stronger (then gotten weaker), built up endurance (then returned to the couch…).

So why change now, and why in such a public way? If everybody has something wrong, why not just live with my problem?

It's not a simple answer, but some of you will understand this statement…*it was just time*. It really cannot be described, but it was just one of those moments in life where in my mind I was done fighting. It was time to do something, anything. Time to get my life where it was supposed to be.

In short, I'd dressed up my problem in a nice little package of excuses for far too long, and now it was time to get undressed.

*"Ladies and Gentlemen, I want to thank you for your patience,"
said the man. "We know these weeks have been stressful with lots
of waiting and wondering. You've all been through a lot to this
point, and you're wanting to know what happens next."*

*"Well, unfortunately, you all need to get in touch with your
families tonight... and let them know you may not be home for
quite a long time..."*

*With this statement the room erupted into laughter,
applause, screams, and tears. Everyone jumped up from his
or her seats and suddenly total strangers were hugging and
high-fiving. The anxiety was instantly gone, and there was a
joy and excitement that took over each of us. Finally, we could
talk and we began introducing ourselves to one another. There
were people from Michigan (lots of them), others from Indiana,
California, Virginia, Missouri, Georgia, and Washington DC. I
began to realize that we were going to get to experience life with
a diverse group of Americans.*

*I looked at Chism and said, "I cannot believe we made it!"
We hugged and celebrated. We began the process of letting
everything soak in. However, as I sat back down, I began to
think, "Oh no, I cannot believe we made it... I might not be home
for a while. What about my family? My job? My ministry?" This
seemed really cool until right this second. What was I thinking?
What is God doing with me?*

*Everybody's got something, and suddenly I realized my
something was about to be on display for millions of people to
see. The real adventure was about to begin.*

A Plan and a Purpose

I mentioned that I often thought of my weight issue as my
thorn in my flesh. It was just my "something" to deal with, like

Paul dealt with the thorn in his flesh. The thing most people forget about Paul is that he prayed for help. He did not like his thorn *or* use it as an excuse. He asked God to remove it and when He did not, Paul then let God use this weakness to show Christ's strength. **Paul's thorn was a tool for God's plan not an excuse for Paul's selfishness.**

This was where God began to change my thinking. I'd held onto and embraced my weight issues because I was unwilling and often afraid to let them go. I didn't want to fail one more time. My poor health was my "something," and I planned to suffer with it for the rest of my life. But maybe, just maybe, my "something" was something God wanted to use, and He was *waiting* for me to ask Him for help. So I offered my issue, the issue of my health, to God. I asked Him to help me get better and to use it for His purposes… Obviously, I had no idea what I was asking.

Undressing Your Something

Now here is the tough part: you have to figure out what *your* "something" is. What do you tolerate or accept as just a part of life because you are honestly just unwilling or afraid to let it go? For me, it was my health, and maybe that's it for you as well. But maybe it's something totally different. My guess is that even as you are reading these words, you already know what it is. It's not typically something hidden, we are fully aware of it. So give your something a name (out loud) and ask God to help you get better and use it for His purposes.

Here's the awesome part. Our big God has something unbelievable in store for you if you are willing to sacrifice your "something." Maybe you cannot imagine life without your "something" always being there, but I can promise you that there is a great life ahead, but only if you let God have it and use it for His purposes. It starts with offering it up and being willing to let it go.

Once you accept the fact that everyone has issues to be addressed, then change is able to happen. You are not alone. We all have things to address. While many will continue to make excuses for their "thing" or try to keep hiding it, how about you start today addressing what needs to be undressed from you?

MAIN POINTS TO REMEMBER

- **You're ready to change.**

  Maybe you aren't sitting in a hotel room of a reality show, but you have obviously arrived at a place where you are ready to make some changes, or you wouldn't be reading this book.

- **Be open to the fact that your 'something' might be a symptom of an underlying problem.**

  As I said, our problem isn't usually hidden, but sometimes the part of it we can see is really identifying an underlying problem. Be ready to address issues you need to fully undress.

- **God wants to use your something for a purpose that you don't yet see.**

  Remember to see your problem as a challenge that God is going to use in your life. Don't view it as an excuse to keep living life the way you have been up to this point. No more saying, "Well, everyone has something . . . I guess this is mine"

Questions for discussion or thought

1. Everybody has "something". What is your something?

2. Why do you suppose it is so difficult for us to address our issues? Do you find yourself attacking your "something" or making excuses for it?

3. If God would help you make a change in this area of your life, what would you like to see yourself do? Dream big!

4. What is the number one thing that is keeping you from removing this obstacle from your life right now?

CHAPTER 3

Redefining Relationship

"Treasure your relationships, not your possessions."

– Anthony J. D'Angleo

Loneliness is terrible. If you've ever been in a situation where you felt truly alone, then you know what I mean. Sometimes I enjoy being by myself (and I even think I can do it longer than many), but I always reach a point where I just have to interact with people.

I experienced some of the deepest moments of loneliness through my experience on The Biggest Loser. There were times when I would lie in my bed writing letters home with tears rolling down my face. In those moments, I felt the pain of homesickness and loneliness like never before. Yes, I understand that God is always there, and I am never truly alone; I know this is true and believe it. However, the moments where I sat in my room and realized that nobody on the other side of my bedroom door truly knew me were quite literally painful.

Pain in our body is used to warn us that something is

wrong. The pain of loneliness is no different. It tells us that something is wrong, something we can't ignore.

And We Being Many, Are One

My favorite "behind the scenes" story I tell began the second week on the show. Buddy, a fellow contestant and pastor from Michigan (which you will hear much more about through this book), and I were visiting, and he brought up an idea, "What if we did church?" Exploring this thought further we decided to meet every Sunday evening, when there was typically no filming. Once workouts were finished for the day we planned to just share and pray with each other. After bouncing it around a little between us, we discussed the idea with some of the other contestants. We decided to give it a try. Out of those talks "BLurch" (Biggest Loser Church) was born…

The first week we met, there were six or seven of us. I shared a little from the Bible and talked for a minute about encouraging each other through this journey. Buddy then opened the door for people to share ways we could pray for each other. We closed our time praying for one another, gave hugs and went to bed. I thought it was awesome, but I was not sure what others thought.

In the weeks to come, I got my answer. During the next week and the weeks to follow, most of the contestants were there. They did not want to miss this time together. Within a couple of weeks, even our production assistants and staff members of the show who stayed with us were attending regularly. About eight weeks in, we actually had a baptism in the pool! Everyone came, shared their thoughts, and was encouraged.

Now you need to understand, not all of us believed the same thing. In fact, we discovered later that the reason so many initially came was that they were afraid there would be "strategy" discussions, and they did not want to be talked about or potentially "voted out." But even when they realized the time together had nothing to do with the show, they still came.

Some were Christians from different denominations. We had a couple of agnostics (God is there but He doesn't care), some with a Jehovah's Witness background, and atheists...but they all came, and we all enjoyed this time together. This was the most unique church I had ever been a part of. I remember a person saying during a prayer time, "I do not really believe in prayer, but since you are going to do it anyway would you pray for my back?" I had never heard that level of honesty in all my years in the church!

One week, as we were about to start, one person said, "Before you begin I just want you to know that I think Jesus was a great person in history, but I don't believe he was God's son, and I don't believe the Bible is God's Word. I don't even think it can be trusted as an accurate historical book." At this, he stopped and just waited for a reply. I remember Buddy and I looking at one another and realizing that God was changing what we had planned for the night. We simply started asking questions about what he thought and this brought out other questions from the others in the room. It ended up being an amazing time of discussion for the whole group. Can you imagine how this might have been received in our typical churches today?

I very quickly found myself really loving these people and wanting the best for their lives. Our church time together was the one time a week we were all able to put the reality TV stuff to the side and just share our hearts and lives with one another. We had tapped into the incredible truth that God had made us to live in community. We each genuinely desired to connect and relate with others.

It was interesting to learn, after the fact, that other shows and other seasons have had this same thing occur. Desire for connection and relationship seems to come to the surface despite the environment of competition. People are hardwired to share life with others, and in spite of our best efforts to remain independent, the truth is evident; we need each other.

We All Want to Matter to Someone

Despite our best efforts to convince others that we can make it on our own, the truth is, feeling alone is terrible. We all desire attention and acceptance no matter how much some of us may try to convince ourselves, and others, that we do not. I learned a number of years ago that there are three levels of attention that people seek:

Positive Attention: *This is what happens when we are in a crowd of people that know and like us. We fit in, and we feel good in this environment because we are getting attention that encourages us and feeds us. Everyone strives for this.*

Negative Attention: *We experience this when we are in the crowd, but we have differences of opinion or lifestyle. Surprisingly, this level of attention is not terrible. While interacting with people who do not agree with us can be stressful, at least we are getting attention. And that's certainly better than no attention at all.*

No Attention: *Being in the midst of a crowd and feeling like no one even notices you are there is one of the worst experiences to have. It is the depth and definition of* *true loneliness. To live life this way usually begins with denial (I do not need anybody anyway!) and leads to despair (I'll just settle for anybody who acknowledges me).*

The interesting part is the thought behavior we see in each level:

- **People who get positive attention are the least open to change.**

  When we receive positive attention and are among a group of people we consider friends, we desire to stay there (of course) and will often do whatever it takes to maintain this status *and the level of comfort that comes with it.* Change is scary and hard because it threatens our comfort level and therefore might threaten our attention status. (In the example of poor physical habits, if we are among friends who love us as we are, we can convince ourselves that we don't need to change.)

- **People who get negative attention are more open to change.**

  When we get negative attention, we tend to want to either move towards a middle ground or help people to embrace our way of thinking. Change is not as scary because our ultimate goal is to get attention with the hope of moving toward a more positive type of attention. (We had a girl on the show that was always getting negative attention by being disagreeable or trying to get people to embrace her way of thinking. Ultimately, she was just trying to belong and had to discover that about herself before she could change.)

- **People who get no attention tend to be the most open to change.**

  People who feel like they get no attention will do anything to get some. Even if it means getting negative attention, they figure at least it's attention. Change is welcome because it can be used as a "shared experience" that gives us something to relate with others about. (It's why we see groups like Alcoholic's Anonymous work so well, because everyone shares their same negative experience and in doing so, begins to feel like part of a community, ultimately longing for positive attention from their peers.)

We see and deal with this all our lives, and at different times experience different levels. No matter what, one thing is consistent: *nobody wants to feel neglected or alone, ever.* Simply put, we were created to desire community. We want to connect with others, preferably in a positive way, but we will settle for the negative if it keeps us in some kind of contact with other people.

The One Another Factor

None of this is an accident. We are told, right in the beginning of the Bible, that we are made in the likeness of God. Our desire to relate to others exists so that we can be reminded that He desires to relate to us. **We are not God's reality show**.

He did not create this planet and then throw us on it so He could sit back and watch. Our yearning for attention mirrors His. We are here to relate with Him and with one another.

Try this, go to an online Bible (I prefer www.youversion.com) and type "one another" in the search. Then take some time to explore all the ways this phrase is used. Here are a few examples:

- be devoted to one another

- challenge one another

- greet one another

- be hospitable to one another

- bear one another's burdens

- discuss with one another

- love one another

It is clear that we are to live life with one another. So it is no surprise that when 20 strangers are thrown into a stressful ever-changing environment and an opportunity to connect in a positive way is presented to them, they do respond. I call it the "one another" factor. We were made for one another. There's no escaping it and no escaping the responsibility that comes with it.

I remember when one of the other contestants came to Buddy and me and asked a really interesting question. "Do you really want to have church? Don't you want a break?" I do not think I completely understood what they were asking, so they elaborated. "Well, all of us here are getting time away from our job. Whether it is retail, medical, banking, etc. we do not have to think about our jobs while we are here." They continued, "You guys are pastors, so as long as we have church, you are still having to work. Don't you want a break too?"

Truthfully, I had to think about this for a bit before realizing my answer. I told them, "Relating with people and connecting all of us with Christ is not my job; it is my life. It feeds me and honestly, it is probably the only thing that is keeping me sane!"

I realized something I seemed to have forgotten. I love people. Getting to know people is not something I do because I have to. Loving others is part of who I am. This defines an important issue for all of you seeking true health in all areas of your life. To be really healthy, you must give up the "me vs. the world" mentality. We are meant to live in relationship. Where you are strong I may be weak, and where you are weak I might be strong. This is the way we were created; it's in our DNA. We need each other and by learning to relate we make life healthier for the both of us.

Living in Community Requires Us to Be Honest

As we neared the end of the show, something happened that I do not think those in charge saw coming, we became incredibly close to one another. Sharing this experience and the struggle we encountered crossed over team or trainer lines to develop strong bonds with one another.

While we were there, we had the amazing opportunity to go to Hawaii, something I had always dreamed of. While we were all longing for family to be there with us, we enjoyed sharing the trip with each other. None of us had ever been, so we became family and soaked in this beautiful place together.

Early on, it was apparent to me that one of the contestants who had become a good friend, Kim, was not really happy or connected. Through circumstances of the politics of game play, she felt isolated, and it was really obvious. She and I had become great competitors and because of our friendship it was hard for me to watch her miss this experience due to some anger and paranoia about what might happen next.

It would have been easy to just "let her be," but that just did not sit right with me. So in a down moment between filming, I took time to encourage her and let her know she mattered and challenged her to enjoy where we all were. She needed to know that someone was on her side.

The change in her was almost instantaneous. I watched her begin to savor not only the trip, but also everything about the relationships with others. Most interestingly, her new attitude continued even once we returned to the ranch. She just needed to know she mattered and once she felt assured that she did, everything was different for her. To this day, she tells people I am like her brother. At its core, this is the purpose of our call to relate to one another, because people matter to God and therefore should matter to us.

We Are an Example to the People in our Lives

How I've regarded my health and fitness has not just affected my life but also the lives of so many around me. While I should not take the blame for other people's choices, I have to own my responsibility in this. If I truly believe that our bodies are unique and special creations of God, not only should I take care of mine, but I must also challenge others to take care of theirs. And as their pastor, mentor, teacher, friend, (insert label here), I have to remember that I am also an example. My actions count for something.

MAIN POINTS TO REMEMBER

- **You weren't created to live life alone.**

  If you really want to be healthy then you must stop thinking it's you against the world. You were created to need others. Your strengths help my weaknesses, and your weaknesses are overcome by my strengths. We were made for each other; it's hard-wired into us. We need each other and by learning to relate we make life healthier for the both of us.

- **We have to be honest and vulnerable.**

  When we truly care for others, when we embrace real relationship, we have to be willing to be honest with the people in our lives. Sure, it's risky. It makes us vulnerable and might cause us to fear being rejected. But imagine what might have happened if I hadn't taken that risk with Kim?

- **Our actions are an example.**

  We have to remember that as we work on ourselves, we are also being used to work in the lives of others. You are ready to make this change in your life, and as you do this for yourself, you are doing it for others as well. Keep moving forward and get ready for the unexpected reward that comes from connecting with others in this life.

Questions for discussion or thought

1. What is the purpose of relationships in your life? Be honest, is it more about what they do for you or what you do for them?

2. Describe the kind of person you are. Do you like having lots of relationships in your life or just a few, deeper ones? Are you outgoing or do you tend to keep to yourself?

3. How likely are you to look for ways to connect with other people? Why do you or why don't you?

4. Do you believe God has placed in you something He wants to use in the lives of others? If so, what do you think that could be?

CHAPTER 4

Twenty Strangers

"Nothing is perfect. Life is messy. Relationships are complex. Outcomes are uncertain. People are irrational."

– Hugh Mackay

It was revealed pretty quickly that living with total strangers while under the lens of a TV camera was going to be rough. Twenty people. That is how many made the final roster...twenty. Out of the thousands that went to open casting calls, and the tens of thousands who applied and sent in videos...twenty.

Twenty people. Twenty hurting people, strangers with very different backgrounds, forced together in an incredibly stressful setting.

Twenty people who had all gotten themselves into the same situation, and were now being given the opportunity of a lifetime to make changes; an opportunity that others could only dream of receiving. Look at the make-up of our group: a father/son from Texas, a mother/daughter from Maryland and another one from Missouri, a 5th grade teacher, an ex-wrestler/single mom from Georgia, (yes, I said an ex-wrestler/single mom) an aspiring young writer and her grandmother from Michigan, two stepbrothers…one from California and one from New York who never really got to know each other growing up, another set of brothers also from Michigan, a couple of sets of brothers and sisters from Michigan and Illinois, and rounding out the crew a husband and wife from Indiana (who looked a lot more like they came from the North Pole!) We were different in so many ways, and yet we had one huge thing in common.

Let me take a moment and be really transparent with you. I did not go into this experience to make new friends or build relationships. As far as I was concerned, this was going to be good for my son and me, period. And if sharing it with the other random contestants from all over America would make the process more fun, then great. But these people were strangers. They had their lives, and I had mine. We would spend these fleeting days and weeks together (or months as it turned out for some of us) and then go our separate ways, healthy acquaintances (maybe) but nothing more. However, now I realize how unrealistic that thought was.

You see, I thought I was in control. I had somehow convinced myself that I was in charge. I had my goals and expectations for this experience. But it became overwhelmingly apparent very quickly that things were completely out of my control.

Looking back it is pretty sad that my mind was not in a better place. Do not get me wrong, I had spent lots of time praying through this opportunity really asking God to do a great work in me and also through me. In my own arrogance though, I was thinking more about the overall impact of the show, not the influence and connection of those who would be with me day in and day out. God was not only putting these people with me so I could show His love and grace, He placed them

38

there so they could help me as well. Each of us walked into this experience with unique gifts and talents that were needed. We were a very unique mix, but a handpicked mix; handpicked not by producers but by God.

You Can Pick Your Friends (Or Can You?)

Most of the time the people who come and go in your life are out of your control. You don't get to pick your parents and you have no say in who are your sisters/brothers/aunts/uncles/etc. You sort of pick your friends, usually from an environment that you didn't get to choose. And on some level you choose your spouse…assuming they choose you. Ultimately, many relationships that you have are given to you, not requested by you.

There is a great part of Scripture in James 2 which says, "My dear brothers and sisters, how can you…favor some people over others? For example, suppose someone comes into your meeting dressed in fancy clothes and expensive jewelry, and another comes in who is poor and dressed in dirty clothes. If you give special attention and a good seat to the rich person, but you say to the poor one, "You can stand over there, or else sit on the floor"—well, doesn't this discrimination show that your judgments are guided by evil motives? Basically we are told that everyone matters and we shouldn't try to manipulate which people we think are important.

What's interesting to me is that this principle finds itself in Scripture because it was an issue for people then just as it's an issue for us. We want to think we are in control of our relationships and we want to choose those we think will benefit us the most. However, it seems we learn from this that when we try to maintain control, we actually accomplish the opposite of our desires. The people in your life are there because they are supposed to be.

When I think back on all this, it messes with my brain quite a bit. How often do we try to avoid others whom we know do not really line up with what we believe? My guess is pretty often. As a pastor, one would think that I would have been out there, in the world, connecting, reaching out…but I wasn't. In fact, I did not even **want** to reach out and connect. I was comfortable in my world, and that included those early days on the show. But God was about to rock my world.

I have to say that if I had handpicked a group of people who were going to help Chism and me overcome our struggle with weight, I probably wouldn't have picked very many of those twenty strangers. Many of them had totally different belief systems than mine. They were from different lifestyles, different stages of life, different in just about as many ways as a group of people can be different. Other than our desire to lose weight and get healthier, we seemingly had nothing in common as far as I could see. But God knew I needed them as much as He knew they needed me. And I don't think I could have ever imagined the impact we would have on each other.

When we all met, none of us had any idea what was in store for us. Of course, we all wanted to lose weight and get healthier, but I do not think any of us really knew the impact each person would have. Even now we are not contestants from a TV show; in a weird way we are family. In a very real, true sense of the word…family.

Life in the Bubble

As I said in Chapter 3, we are made to relate, created to connect with others. First, we are to spend time getting to know God through Christ, but then we are to invest in others; not just for what we think we have to offer them, but also for what they can do for us. God has put each of us here in this unique experience called life to get to know one another. The worlds we create are what cause problems. When we seek to live in our own little bubbles, we then develop opinions and prejudices of others who are living in different bubbles. We get comfortable and even begin to believe that our way is the only way that is right.

Now, I am not talking about developing a relationship with God. Scripture makes it incredibly clear that there is only one way to the Father and that is through the gift of His Son, Jesus. What I am referring to are the lives we create for ourselves, often outside the will of God, because those lives make us feel comfortable. Living for others often means allowing us to be interrupted by the needs of the people around us, and stepping away from our own comfort.

One of the greatest examples of giving up our own desire for comfort to meet the needs of others came from my close friend and fellow contestant, Buddy. In his journey to health, he made the difficult decision to trust God with his family back at home, a family that included three small children and one on the way. His amazing wife, Shelby, insisted that he travel down this road, even though it meant she would have to handle things at home while enduring the difficulties of pregnancy. This was so difficult for Buddy, and yet I watched him battle his emotions daily as he pushed forward.

One of the team challenges we won brought a much-cherished reward, a video meeting with our family at home. Homesickness was one of the most difficult parts of the experience, so any chance to connect with family was worth more than gold. However, since Chism and I were on separate teams, the win meant I would get to see our family, and he would not. I knew he needed that motivation so I gave my prize to him. It was hard but it was important for me to let him have this moment.

As we were being interviewed later, I was asked why I would give up this valuable prize for Chism. I simply told them that it was a no-brainer. It was the kind of thing a father should be willing to do for his son. I felt it was just the thing he needed to keep moving forward through this crazy experience.

However, there was a surprise coming that I never expected. The interviewer changed focus to Buddy. I was overwhelmed to hear that when Buddy heard that I sacrificed my prize for Chism, he then chose to sacrifice his prize for me! Chism and I were going to be allowed to have a video chat with our family together. My emotions overtook me, and I was unbelievably humbled by Buddy's selfless decision.

It was instantly clear what this meant for Buddy though, he would not be able to see or communicate with his family. I really struggled with this. For me to give up my prize for my son was one thing, but for Buddy to sacrifice his for me really made no sense. Only weeks earlier we were two of twenty strangers, so for him to give up something so unbelievably valuable was one of the most unexpected gifts of kindness I had ever received.

True Healing Is Found in Community

It took me a while to understand that Buddy "got it." He saw the value of living in community and throwing away one's personal desires for comfort. He was (and is) a living representation of what living for others really looks like.

What Buddy did still stirs emotion in me. He "showed" his love for me by giving up the comfort of seeing his family, a comfort he so desperately needed. He didn't get to choose me as a fellow contestant, roommate, or team member; but he did choose me as a friend.

His sacrifice is such a beautiful example of selflessness and is an incredible picture of the sacrifice Jesus made for each of us. Jesus gave up comfort for the good of all of us because we are that important to Him. It is His example that we are called to follow. We were never designed to live hidden lives in our self-made bubble of comfort. People are important, and I have learned that life in community is where real relationships exist. And it's in real community with God and others that we find healing.

So many parts of this life are beyond our power, but one very important thing is under our control…we get to choose how we treat others. And this one thing can make all the difference.

MAIN POINTS TO REMEMBER

- **Don't be too quick to size up the people God puts in your path.**

  (No pun intended.) We are so quick to judge and dismiss people just because they are different than we are. If I never allowed those twenty strangers to be in my life, I wouldn't have experienced the change that God had for me, physically, emotionally, and spiritually.

- **Sometimes what is best for you is not necessarily the thing you would have chosen for yourself.**

  Even though your tendencies lead you one direction, that which is going to truly be part of a healthy life is in another place. Part of the joy in living is in finding value in every person that enters your life.

- **God wants us to live outside our bubbles and engage in the world around us.**

  When we truly begin to live outside our bubbles, we become less focused on ourselves, and more focused on the needs of others.

Questions for discussion or thought

1. Do you agree that you don't really choose the people who intercept your life? Why or why not?

2. People today seem to be more and more focused on their small world. Do you think this is true? Why or why not?

3. Are you someone who willingly gives up comfort for the good of others? How do you feel when others interrupt your plans?

4. "We are made to relate. We are created to connect with others." Do you agree with this statement? Why or why not?

CHAPTER 5

Removing Fear

"I have learned over the years that when one's mind is made up, this diminishes fear; knowing what must be done does away with fear."

– Rosa Parks

Most people have had this dream. You leave your home, you are out in public – maybe a store or a classroom— and suddenly you realize you are not wearing anything. The dream usually involves running around trying to get away from people or hoping to find something to cover yourself, but you never get covered and people are looking and laughing. Even when you wake up from the dream, it takes a few minutes to fully recover as you realize it was not real, and no one has actually seen you undressed.

But what happens if it's not a dream?

There was a lot of excitement about being on television and the life change that was ahead. We were excited for all the things to come, but there was one moment just around the corner that we were dreading. The first episode on The Biggest

Loser is always the same; at some point all of the contestants must walk up to the famous scale and let the world see what they have done to themselves. And the twenty of us would be no different, our moment was just around the corner. For overweight people there is nothing quite as fearful as being seen with your shirt off, and we were about to do it in front of millions of viewers.

I still remember the day. There was some comfort in knowing I was going to experience this with others who were in the same boat. But when that moment came for me to stand there alone, facing everyone else in the room, I thought I might pass out. This was not "normal" to me. Lights, cameras, and an audience of millions of unknown people were all in front of me as I took off my shirt and waited to see what the numbers would say. It was humbling, embarrassing, and painful...but at the same time it was healing.

After the first time, the fear just seemed to dissipate. Each week got better, and as I saw physical improvement, the fear was quieted. Facing my fear of public humiliation was not to be the only fear I would battle during my time on The Biggest Loser. There were many, including the fear of the unknown, fear of losing control, fear of losing my reputation, and even the fear of losing my faith and disappointing God.

Excuses, Excuses, Excuses

Pretty much every single person I have ever spoken to about health and fitness issues knows *what* to do about their problem, and even how to get started, but much like people who struggle with any issue, they are filled with excuses as to why they can't do it.

I don't say that in a harsh way. I get it. I struggled for years with my weight and overall health. Excuses make it easy to face ourselves in the mirror each day. But excuses are often just lies we have convinced ourselves are truth.

I recently took the opportunity to poll people on my Facebook page about what is "the" excuse that keeps them from choosing to be healthy. The bulk of the responses looked like this:

- I am too tired…
- I like food too much…
- I'm not motivated…
- I do not have time…
- It is too expensive…

In total, there were 30 written responses. What is interesting is that 830 people viewed the question, which means 800 did not even respond. Most did not want to *address* the issue with an answer, possibly because in answering the question, they were admitting they had an excuse. I wonder if I had asked, "What is one thing that keeps you from getting healthy?" if more people would have answered.

Funny thing is, when we label something as a "reason" we can convince ourselves it's okay. But once we label it an excuse, we know we have to deal with it.

As I looked through the list of excuses people gave, I recognized the root of those excuses as the same root of my own excuses: fear.

- **I am too tired** can mean I don't have the energy to try, and I'm afraid I'll only fail (again).
- **I like food too much** can mean I like my foods too

much, and I am afraid I will not like the healthy stuff.

- **I do not have motivation** can mean I do not see the importance of trying, and I am afraid it will be a waste of effort.

- **I do not have time** can mean I do not see my health as a priority, and I am afraid of what adding one more thing to my schedule would mean.

- **It is too expensive** can mean I don't think I can focus on my health without spending more money, and I'm afraid it will all end up being for nothing.

Facing Down Fear

Fear can be crippling and is one of the biggest tools the enemy uses to keep us from accomplishing what God has placed us on earth to do.

I mentioned the fears I battled on the show:

Fear of the unknown (or fear of not being in control)

I did not like the unknown, I was constantly afraid of what they would throw at us next... and what they threw at us next was pretty much constant 24/7 change. How could I prepare for what I do not foresee? However, as I faced this fear, I began to learn that God does not have to show me His plan. In fact, His plan for me, the next thing around the corner, is probably so much bigger than I can imagine that I am not sure I would join Him if I knew how big His plan really was.

Fear of losing my reputation

It is scary being vulnerable in any environment, much less one where you are completely out of control. I know how reality shows like to use the editorial process to create the "reality" they want to create. What if my reputation wasn't maintained or portrayed accurately?

Fear of losing my faith or disappointing God

My life had been spent within the confines of the "Christian" world, surrounded by fellow Christ-followers in a safe environment. Stepping out of this was hard and frightening...what if my faith collapsed?

Every single day I had to face and battle the fear that had gotten me in this situation in the first place.

Driven by Fear

Recently I was looking at John 18, where Jewish leaders take Jesus to the Roman governor. I've always been fascinated with this story, repeated by all four of the gospel writers. It's interesting to note that the fact that Jesus was handed over for judgment and eventually death is never disputed. You will likely never find people arguing that Jesus was an innocent man who was violently killed. Biblical and non-biblical writers agree on this truth. But how in the world did this story escalate so dramatically? One word: fear.

The religious leaders had their way of life. They held to many rules that gave them comfort in their faith. Anyone who came along and threatened to shake up the comfort structure immediately created fear. The religious leaders were waiting for the Messiah, but they wanted him under their terms, and wanted him to meet their expectations. Jesus did neither.

What is interesting is that when you look at this passage, the leaders were taking Him to the Roman governor's palace and it says, "His accusers did not go inside because it would defile them, and they would not be allowed to celebrate Passover." Look at what is being said here! Apparently walking into the palace would have violated some religious requirement, but assisting in the murder of an innocent man did not.

This is such an amazing picture of how far they were willing to go because of fear and they never even saw it in themselves. If Jesus were truly who He said He was, then they knew everything would have to change. And their fear of change, their fear of the unknown, their fear of losing control, it all led to an unfair trial filled with lies and ultimately to Jesus' death.

Change can be hard, it can hurt; routines take a long time to develop and there is a level of comfort in them. Fear rears its head whenever we see anything that may challenge our routine. At some point though, we must be convinced that life on the other side of the fear is better.

I love this verse, "There is no fear in love; but perfect love casts out fear, because fear involves punishment, and the one who fears is not perfected in love," 1 John 4:18. This reminds me that love comes first; God's love for me, my love for others and myself. But it also tells me that love trumps the fear; fear of failure, fear of change, fear of trying one more time.

I Can Do All Things

On our first night we had a three-part challenge that determined who would make it on the show and who would not. It began with a 40-yard dash…not too hard, right? Chism and I decided that I would run for our team. I was glad to run, and I weighed less than any of the guys who were there. All I had to do was make it in the top 4 and we would secure a place on the ranch. I was extremely nervous but very confident that I could do well.

The run started, and I was able to get ahead of everyone for a second. The finish line was not too far away so things looked promising until "it" happened.

The show's medical trainer called it my "sniper shot," and from the pain, I figured it was a good description. About halfway through the run, I felt an intense pain shoot through my left hamstring. I could not keep my balance and ended up having an absolutely beautiful and acrobatic fall on the path. As soon as I hit the ground, it was clear something was really wrong. Once I stood up and started to walk, I realized I was in trouble. This was not the way to start this experience.

Turns out in a simple 40-yard dash, my hamstring tore. My workouts had to be modified and right from the start my journey began to look differently than I had planned. I had not even made it to the first workout, and I was already injured. This was not good.

I found out later that some of the others were questioning my injury. Some were not sure I was hurt at all and thought it was just a ploy so that I did not have to do the same level of workouts as everyone else. My disappointment and discouragement were at an all time high. I no longer wanted to do any of this. I just wanted to go home.

Chism and I talked over the next week, and I began to prepare his mind for what to do if I was not there. I still wanted him to get the most he could out of this, but I had convinced myself that I was on my way out. Every day brought new fear about whether I could or would actually succeed. It was very *easy to imagine just giving up and going back to what was comfortable. The fear was urging me to head back to the life I understood, even though it was not a healthy life, at least it was a life that made sense.*

However, God had other plans. First off, I just could not get sent home! Either my team would win or I would do so well that my leaving was not an option. The relationships I had formed became more valuable to me than the idea of running away to my perceived comfort at home. The impact of fear was decreasing on my daily life.

Another thing that was happening was that God was changing my attitude about the fear. As I began to see success, it became clearer that fear's bark was very often worse than its bite. Physically, mentally, emotionally, and spiritually, I was getting stronger and fear became a challenge that I wanted to overcome, not an emotion that drove me away from the task. God was working on and in me to remove the power that fear had over me, and in typical "God fashion", He did it in a way and a place that I would have never expected, The Biggest Loser ranch.

Do not let fear win. Be willing to let go and see what life is like when our fears are addressed and removed. God has something better for us on the other side of the fear, but the only way to step forward is to be overwhelmed by His love. Choose not to be overcome by fear, but instead boldly walk into your healthy life covered by His love today.

MAIN POINTS TO CONSIDER

- **Most excuses are born of fear.**

  Remember that excuses are lies born of fear, and both are tools the enemy uses to keep us from accomplishing our purpose in life, our God-given purpose.

- **Fear limits motivation.**

  The body has an autonomic response to real fear (a response placed in our bodies by God). It's called fight or flight. It dumps a crazy amount of adrenaline and dopamine into our bodies, which tell us either to stand and fight, or to run away. Notice that neither of our responses to fear should be "give up." It is the fear that the enemy creates in us that limits our motivation to change. Never give up. Use your fear as a source of motivation. Stand and fight!

- **God has a better plan.**

  Release our fears to God and accepting His plan for our life is always the better choice. I'm not saying it's the easier choice. But it's the best one.

Questions for discussion or thought

1. Is there a fear that is continually keeping you from moving forward with your goals? What is it? Where do you believe it comes from?

2. Most of us deal with some kind of fear. So why do you think we still feel like we are the only ones who struggle?

3. It can be hard and scary to experience change in life. What parts of change tend to cause you the most anxiety or fear?

4. Look ahead and imagine the fear wasn't there. What could life look like beyond the fear? How might God use you in the absence of your fear?

CHAPTER 6

Stress Happens

"It is not stress that kills us, it is our reaction to it."

– Hans Selye

Life teaches all of us in various ways. Our different cultures, different backgrounds, and different life experiences all work to shape us into the people we become. You may be very open and outgoing, or you may be reserved and shy. You may be cautious when stepping into new relationships or welcoming to anyone. Some people are great with a group and struggle with individual connection while others may feel socially awkward with many people but have a knack for going deep in one-on-one situations. We hold different motivations, different pains, different joys, and different passions. All of these differences make us unique. There is a reason why I like the phrase, "Be yourself...you're the only one who can be."

Sometimes, though, our "uniqueness" can be a source of struggle and conflict because we also carry our burdens in our own way. Take twenty people from various backgrounds and experiences, highlight their greatest visibly painful issue in front of millions of television viewers, and well, stress happens.

Stress was the one thing we could always count on being present on the show, no matter what we were doing, where we were going, or whom we were meeting, stress was there. And one of my greatest moments of stress on the show has become a story that will likely be passed down through our family for generations to come. Looking back now on the events of that day, I can laugh and retell the story with great dramatic flair. But in the moment, it was probably the most stressful thing I have ever experienced in my life.

Of all the amazing experiences we had during our time on the show, one stands out above the rest. We were given the privilege of being invited to the White House to meet and work out with the First Lady, Michelle Obama. When this news came to us, each of us was speechless. This was an opportunity like none other.

Not only would we be allowed to have this special time at the White House, we would be able to share it with our family. As contestants, this held even more value as it was at the end of the show's famed "makeover week," a week where the remaining participants get to show off their new look to their family after months of hard work...

After traveling across the country, we arrived in Washington D.C., and were escorted to the White House to make our way through security. Even though we had not seen them yet, we knew that somewhere on these special grounds was our family whom we had not seen in months. We were more excited and overwhelmed than words can describe.

We were taken through this landmark home to one of the two massive circular driveways outside. I remember clearly looking at the beautiful house on one side and looking across the huge lawn on the other side where I saw the famous Washington Monument in the distance. Even though it was rainy and a little chilly, there was nothing that could dampen my awe in that moment.

As we were led across the driveway, we noticed a white van similar to the ones that transported us everywhere we went. The only difference was in this van they had placed black curtains on all the windows so that once we were inside, we would be unable to see out. We were all placed in the van and given some simple instructions about what would happen next. Each person would go in, one at a time, to be "revealed." They wanted to capture the emotion on a person-by-person basis. The order was given, and I was to be the last person to be taken inside. That is exactly when my stress began.

Here is where you need a little background information. On days when we filmed, each person had to be accounted for at all times. You not only had to let them know where you were, but you often traveled the grounds with an escort so that someone could find you at a moment's notice. This included going to the restroom. (It was like grade school all over again.) The thing that made this more of an issue was that as we were getting healthier we were learning the need to drink more water; lots of water, all the time. This meant our restroom breaks were a regular occurrence, for some of us more than others. Very often, if you had to "go", it was an interruption to the process, so we tried to plan accordingly. (Sometimes this worked and sometimes not so much.)

Back in the van outside of the White House, I suddenly realized that I had not "taken care of business" and now here I was, stuck in the van, waiting my turn to go in. As I thought about my options, I realized production was rolling and the interruption of a restroom break was going to be significant, certainly compounded by the fact that we were not just in any location. Taking a break would involve pausing the show, as well as connecting with the Secret Service to be escorted to facilities within the White House. Because of the complications that I had established in my mind, I decided to wait it out. After all, how long would I possibly have to sit there anyway?

An hour-and-a-half later, I found myself alone in a white van with blackened out windows on the circular drive of the White House, and I was about to explode. My stress level was at epic proportions. I could not wait any longer, but at that point I would not disturb production, so I got creative.

I began searching under the seats looking for anything that would work to hold some "liquid". Fortunately I found a large cup under the very back seat of the van. I took the cup and moved to the front of the van, got on my knees between the captain's chairs and tried to focus. (Now understand, this was no small feat as I was in a full suit and tie, decked out and ready to go meet the First Lady at any moment)

Then came a knock on the side van door.

Panic hit me, and I scrambled to compose myself. I slowly opened the door and no one was there. In those seconds, as I tried to figure out if I had truly heard a knock, a gloved hand grabbed the door and pulled it open. Standing before me was a Secret Service agent, fully armed and ready to protect our nation's capital from whatever was happening in this van.

The tall, smartly dressed agent politely asked me what I was doing, I explained about the show, and that I was waiting to go in. He looked around the inside of the van, called in to make sure this was okay and then started to walk away. He paused, turned back slowly, and before I closed the door asked, "Sir, are you sure you are alright?" I said yes, and assured him I was fine, at which point he wished me a good day and left.

By then, any desire I had to relieve myself disappeared. My heart rate was pounding at an unbelievable pace, and I decided I could just hang in there. That feeling lasted for about 60 seconds after which it was unbearably obvious that I had not taken care of my problem. It had to be dealt with.

In full panic mode, I quickly grabbed the cup and reassumed my position at the front of the van, relaxing until eventually nature took its course. I reveled in that moment of amazing and instantaneous relief until a thought hit me, "What do I do with this cup now?"

In my panic-driven need to relieve myself, I literally never thought about what I would do afterwards. I was sitting in van, which had already drawn the suspicions of the Secret Service, on the circular driveway of the White House, dressed in a full suit and tie, waiting to meet the First Lady for a nationwide television show I was on...and I was holding a full cup of pee.

What in the world does that story have to do with stress?

Stress hits us from all different directions. Sometimes it's a result of the circumstances of our life, but sometimes it's a result of our own choices. Regardless of the source of our stress, we must identify it and make the conscious decision to let it go.

Now I know that sounds like an over-simplified statement, and some might laugh at the story I used to make the point. But the fact is, we all struggle with stress, and sometimes a thought as simple as "just releasing it" does not make sense. But the truth is, holding on to stress will never make it better—in fact it usually makes it worse. Add into this our attempts to deal with stress on our terms, in our own way, and we often turn a bad situation into an unbearable one.

Stress Management 101

In Matthew 6, Jesus addresses how He wants us to handle the stress and worries that plague us in this world. I've included the entire passage so you can personally read what He has to say on the subject:

> *"Therefore I tell you, do not worry about your life, what you will eat or drink; or about your body, what you will wear. Is not life more than food, and the body more than clothes? Look at the birds of the air; they do not sow or reap or store away in barns, and yet your heavenly Father feeds them. Are you not much more valuable than they? Can any one of you by worrying add a single hour to your life?*

> *"And why do you worry about clothes? See how the flowers of the field grow. They do not labor or spin. Yet I tell you that not even Solomon in all his splendor was dressed like one of these. If that is how God clothes the grass of the field, which is here today and tomorrow is thrown into the fire, will he not much more clothe you—you of little faith? [31] So do not worry, saying, 'What shall we eat?' or 'What shall we drink?' or 'What shall we wear?' [32] For the pagans run after all these things, and your heavenly Father knows that you need them. [33] But seek first his kingdom and his righteousness, and all these things will be given to you as well. [34] Therefore do not worry about tomorrow, for tomorrow will worry about itself. Each day has enough trouble of its own. Matthew 6:25-34 NIV*

In essence He says, "Focus on Me, and I'll take care of the rest." After all, who among us can add a single day to our lives with worry? The answer is none, but as we read in the passage, we can certainly take a few days away if we let stress consume us. In fact, when we deal with stress and try to control things in our own way, without heeding Christ's instructions, we end up more stressed out and with more problems than we had in the first place.

I know that's true of me. Food was my comfort in times of stress. So I convinced myself that I controlled the one thing that had in truth controlled *me* for most of my life. I was deceived. My stress was not being dealt with correctly and looking back, I know I was never in control.

But it's so easy to believe that we are in control, so easy to justify our stress behaviors (and don't kid yourself into thinking that eating is the only destructive behavior people use to manage stress). I often justified my stress eating as a "reward" I gave myself for the good work I was doing for Jesus. Working for God is honorable and good, but it's also incredibly stressful and difficult. I believed that I was entitled to the comfort that food offered as a stress releaser.

In the midst of believing that lie, I lost sight of this truth: focusing only on Jesus and giving Him everything is God's way of dealing with stress.

If He is truly the only thing that matters then there is never a situation or circumstance that He does not have full control over. If He says focus on Me and let Me handle all the other stuff, then He must really be able to handle that stuff without us.

Taking control and trying to deal with stress our own way is sin. We can try to dress it up, but at its core we are saying to God, 'my way is better than Yours."

UNDRESSED

I like how Larry Crabb put it. *"Sin is an attempt to meet a legitimate need in an illegitimate way."* Resolving stress is a legitimate need we have as human beings. But resolving stress with destructive behaviors (like comfort eating) only ends up making us feel worse about ourselves than we did before we took matters into our own hands.

Think about this, if He can take care of it all, that has to be one of the most freeing truths of all time. I do not have to worry. I do not have to let stress control me. That means that I have no need for that "thing" I do to deal with stress.

If He can take care of it all, then we do not have to worry. We do not have to let stress control us. Therefore, we have no need for the behaviors we have created to deal with our stress.

So I was in the most awkward situation I had ever been in. I was sitting in a van, at the White House, holding a cup of my own urine, and completely stressed out. I had to do something and do it quickly.

I made a quick decision and chose to pour it out on the ground by opening the door a little. The rain would help so no one would be suspicious as to why there was a wet spot outside the van. I geared myself up and prepared to do it quickly. However, in a fast burst of adrenaline, I threw the van door wide open and flung the contents of the cup as far as I could get them to fly. After slamming the door I crushed the cup (so that no one would accidentally use it later…) and resumed my waiting. Honestly, I was feeling a little proud of myself until I heard another knock at the van door…

It dawned on me that since I was in a blackened out van I couldn't see who might have been standing around when I sprayed our nation's capital with my DNA. I was ready for a Secret Service agent to pull me out and take me away. I could just imagine the headlines about how a pastor from Texas defiantly poured his urine on the White House lawn as a statement against our government. The stress that had come and gone was back in full force.

Slowly, I opened the door ready for whatever lay ahead and was instantly relieved to see one of our awesome production associates, Kristen. It was time for me to go inside...

On the way to enter this historic building for a once in a lifetime experience, she looked at me and said, "What was up with the Secret Service guy? Why was he bothering you?" I looked at her and simply said, "I have no idea..."

The Better Way

Another great example we see of God's idea of stress management comes from Luke 10. Jesus has come to the home of Martha and is sitting around teaching those in the home. Mary is listening to the words He is saying, but Martha is busy getting everything together for her guests. She comes to a point where she is frustrated at working alone and does not like that Mary is doing "nothing".

Jesus says something so fantastic to her. "You are worried and upset over all these details! There is only one thing worth being concerned about. Mary has discovered it, and it will not be taken from her." In a kind way He says, "Stop stressing out and put your mind on what really matters. Mary has figured it out, and I am not going to chastise her for it."

Now very likely, all the things Martha was doing were good things. She was preparing a dinner for her guests, wanting to be a good hostess by making sure things were ready. But even these "good" things were not the most important things. God knows that there are lots of good things for us to do, but they should never be done at the expense of the best thing. Once we understand this and give our stress to Him, everything changes.

Here's the thing though, you must give Him a chance. Sometimes we want to release only a little bit and see how God handles it. Something I've learned about Him is that He is not into sharing. He wants you to let it all go so that you can fully see Him work. Only then are we able to be free.

Look at it this way, if we try and "help" God in dealing with our stress then chances are when He deals with it, we will want some of the credit. Letting it go allows us to fully focus on Him, lets us completely see Him work, and in the end allows us to recognize and give Him the glory for the work He did alone.

Take it from me and my story of stress, it will always be better once you "let it go".

MAIN POINTS TO REMEMBER

- **Stress happens to everyone.**

  Stress does not care where you came from, what you do for a living, how you were raised, or what you have experienced in life. You will never have a life free from stress. So you must learn how to manage it appropriately.

- **Jesus has a perfect stress-management plan.**

  Jesus has laid it all out for us in His Word. Release control to Him, follow His lead, and trust that He can handle whatever comes our way.

- **Our response to stress often increases the stress we feel.**

  Taking matters into our own hands (sin) is always a bad decision with detrimental results. What you think will bring you comfort, in the end, only makes you more stressed.

Questions for discussion or thought

1. Make a list of the things that cause you the most stress. Put them in order from the highest stress to the lowest.

2. What are the most common ways you deal with stress? Are these good and healthy ways or do these lead to more stress?

3. Describe a time where stress got the best of you. What things made it worse? What ultimately made it better?

4. What is the hardest thing about giving up your worries and stresses to God? Why is this a struggle?

PART TWO

Putting On What's True

CHAPTER 7

Grace First

"I do not at all understand the mystery of grace – only that it meets us where we are but does not leave us where it found us."

– Anne Lamott

I really do not know why I've been one of the millions who tune in for this relatively new genre of entertainment called reality TV. It likely has to do with the idea that these shows are real people, not actors, getting to do some really interesting things, and by watching them, I can escape reality and convince myself I might also be able to do those things.

Because of our personal issues with our health, weight loss reality shows have always been popular with our family, The Biggest Loser being a favorite for many years. We tuned in weekly to love, hate, laugh, and cry with the contestants as they worked to get their lives back. Their stories of life change seemed possible in our lives because they were normal people, just like us. (Of course, in the back of my mind, I always told myself they were only successful because they had the assistance of a miracle show to help them.)

And suddenly, I was one of those people – a reality show contestant.

After we found out we made it, the process began with an official weigh-in at our hotel. I remember getting called to the lobby early in the morning, having no idea what was going on. We entered a small room, stepped on a scale, and then received a small challenge. "This weight is your official starting point. Go back to your room, throw away all the junk food you have, and head to the gym to begin working out. You have taken the first step on this road to a healthier, more fit you."

Chism and I took this challenge somewhat seriously.

Grace First

Something really hit me during this time. Through all the craziness, it became clear that God had a bigger goal for this whole thing than just me losing weight. This was going to affect my family, my life, my ministry – everything - in ways I never saw coming. As I began to let that soak in, I realized something very important . . . Before I could get help or become help for others, it was vital for me to see that God loved me where I was - fat, unhealthy, unhappy, tired . . . Christ accepted me, unconditionally, exactly as I was.

While my experience on the show was going to make me more useful in serving Him, and it would allow me to have a greater impact for the truth of the gospel, it would not make me more pleasing to Him. His love for me was already complete. Recognizing His grace for me was the first step in my full recovery.

I had to accept His grace for me **in all areas of my life** if I was to be used of Him.

Suddenly, the first glimpse of this message became real to me. Every person I would encounter on this journey needed to know this! Each individual I would get to share life with, in or out of this show, needed to hear that they mattered to God, and regardless of where they were on their journey, His grace was there. They didn't have to change a thing about themselves to be accepted and loved by Him. Grace was first.

Why We Can't Accept Grace

This is a difficult concept to grasp. (Remember, I had been a pastor for years and I was just now getting it!) Everything in life teaches us that performance equals acceptance. I have to do well to be received well. Sadly, from what I've seen, even though in our churches we talk about grace quite a bit, I do not know that we really let it permeate our lives fully. I know I did not.

There is a great story in Mark 1 where Jesus has been traveling around the area teaching, connecting and healing people. He meets a man with leprosy who says something really interesting, "If you are willing, you can make me clean." (v. 40, NASB) There is so much here in this statement, but if you look closely you will see an underlying expectation. He does not seem to have a problem with whether or not Jesus CAN make him clean; he's not sure He WILL make him clean.

Honestly, doesn't it seem easier to think that God honors our efforts, even a little? Surely our church attendance, our commitment to read the Bible and prayer, sacrificing or standing up for what's right, avoiding things that are unhealthy physically, mentally, or spiritually, surely those all count for something, right?

Fortunately, while all of these behaviors and disciplines will help *us* grow closer to God, they do not affect His love or acceptance of us, at all. He already loves us completely and wholeheartedly, just as we are. If we could influence Him, even a tiny bit, then that would mean we have some control, no matter how small, over God.

I was one who had been guilty of saying; *"I am good at giving grace to others, but poor at giving it to myself."* Truthfully, from my experience on The Biggest Loser, I've come to realize that I was never really all that good at giving grace to others. I realized that if I could not show grace to myself, then how could I expect to show it to others? Grace had to permeate my life first, so that I could then speak it into the lives of others. Without that firsthand experience, sure, I could show others kindness, forgiveness, or even acceptance, but I could not demonstrate grace.

What Is Grace

To understand this we need to make sure we have a solid definition of what grace really is. Probably this is the best statement of true grace, **"the free and unmerited favor of God."** Look at this:

> *Free – grace costs us nothing, there is no price tag, no fine print; grace is there for the taking, an instant do-over or clean slate with no obligation.*

> *Unmerited – grace is never dependent on anything the person receiving it has done, is doing, or will do; no one deserves it or earns it.*

Favor – *this is simply an act of kindness beyond what is due or what is normal; favor is amazing in and of itself, but combining favor with this next phrase should blow us all away.*

Of God – *the Creator of all things looked at us, His creation, and said, "I want to show them favor. I want them to know grace." Not because of anything in us, but completely because of everything in Him, we receive grace.*

Here is why this matters…the great, loving, powerful Creator of all things, our Father who created you in His own image, looks at you and says, "I want to show you favor. My grace is available to you." If He so willingly offers us grace, then surely we must be willing to accept it for ourselves and show it to others.

It dawned on me as well that the message of grace is a great message for some, but a difficult message for others. For those who do not think they are worthy, who never perform up to life's expectation, the message of grace is a glorious thing. They don't have to worry about performing because God doesn't love us based on our performance.

But for those who have lived life performing and seeking to impress, this message hurts a little. Suddenly all their work and effort seems for nothing. The playing field is leveled, and they realize they are on the same level as those who have done nothing to deserve His love.

It was clear to me that my goal was to communicate the message of grace in what I said and how I acted through this experience. The people I would be sharing my life with would be responsible to figure out how they would receive it. I just had no idea that God had such a variety of people He was about to bring into my life.

We hit the room after our weigh-in and got rid of most of the junk food. We threw away some of it, but decide to finish off some of the "good" stuff. Then we called to reserve a time for the gym in the hotel. After waiting for a while, we were given our gym time. We were told other contestants would be with us but that we were not to talk to them...again.

As we made it to the elevator, we encountered two of the other people; they had to be brothers, but of course we could not ask them. We politely smiled and nodded. I was certain they were doing the same thing we were, checking out the competition.

Suddenly, one of the brothers said, "Rangers fans, huh? Sorry for what's about to happen to your boys tonight!"

(We are die-hard Texas Rangers fans in our home. I like to say we've raised our kids the right way because they love baseball. Texas Rangers baseball. As true fans, we have a collection of Rangers t-shirts and wear them proudly whenever possible. Chism and I were both wearing sweet-looking Texas Rangers shirts.)

This guy was not off to a good start with me, talking when we were not supposed to and trashing my Texas Rangers as well. I kindly smiled even though I did not want to and thought about the fact that my "boys" were playing the Tigers that night. This was one of those Michigan people. I should have known...

After our barely intense 20-minute workout, we headed back to the room. Once there, I said to Chism, "Could you believe the attitude of that guy in the elevator? What a jerk! Talking about the Rangers, who does he think he is? We cannot talk to each other, we are about to share a TV show with this guy, and that's how he starts the relationship?"

Fast forward to the first day at "the ranch". Each couple was given a room with a bathroom, their place to call home. Pretty decent accommodations, but ours was especially nice. Our room had TWO bedrooms with a bathroom. Each of the rooms was separated by a single door and held two twin-sized beds. It looked like Chism and I would have our own rooms! We began making plans for pushing the beds together and figuring out who got what room until we heard a knock at our door.

It was the brothers. The trash talker, the rule breaker... the roommates. I was polite, but in my mind I was thinking, "Seriously?" In an instant, we had gone from being excited about having two rooms for just the two of us, to suddenly having two rooms for the four of us. What made matters worse, in my mind, was that of all the potential roomies we could have had, we ended up with these guys. (On a side note, I figured out later, with our starting weights, our room represented just over 1450 lbs. Needless to say we were in tight quarters and our bathroom was pulling double duty...again, no pun intended).

Something in my mind thought, "grace first." God knew what He is doing. There was a plan and a purpose to everything that had happened up to that point. Nothing had been by accident. He had put all this in motion for His glory, so these guys were a part of His plan as well. I needed to show grace first because there was likely a time coming soon where I would need grace from them.

As I took time to get to know these guys, I found that the trash talker, Buddy, was also a pastor. We shared incredibly similar views and a passion for grace and helping others know Jesus. Our friendship on the show was, as Buddy would say, "a normal friendship on crack. You cannot help but get incredibly close, incredibly fast." He became, and still is, one of the closest friends I have ever had.

This relationship, and others, could not have formed, if

we both had not had grace first. In fact, relationships that are formed outside of grace are formed in selfishness. If you connect with someone because of what they do for you that is selfish, but if you bond with someone who offers you nothing in return, that's grace. It's either one way or the other, there is no middle ground.

In our circumstances, I had nothing to offer Buddy, and he had nothing to offer me. We were both messed up with the same problem: pastors who loved their families deeply but had let an issue, their "something," affect their ability to love and serve God. A friendship formed in the strangest of places with the best of origins...grace.

This was just the beginning for us though. Looking back, neither of us could have ever imagined the journey God still had for us ahead.

MAIN POINTS TO REMEMBER

- **God loves you just as you are.**

  There is nothing you can do to earn more of God's love. He is madly in love with you, just as you are right now.

- **God wants you to accept His grace.**

  We can "understand" that God's love for us is not based on our performance, but until we truly "accept" that grace and stop trying to earn His favor, we cannot show grace to others.

- **God wants you to show grace to others.**

  We were created in the image of God. And as we grow closer to Him, we will begin to act more and more like Him. His first act of love toward us is grace, and He wants us to show that same grace to others.

Questions for discussion or thought

1. What does "grace" mean to you? What role has it played in your life to this point?

2. When was there a time that you showed grace to someone else? How did that experience make you feel?

3. Is it easier to show grace to others or to yourself? Why?

4. Is there an area in your life where you need to accept the gift of grace? What is keeping you from receiving it?

CHAPTER 8

God Matters

"Sir, my concern is not whether God is on our side; my greatest concern is to be on God's side, for God is always right."

– Abraham Lincoln

*M*y best and worst day on the show happened back to back. There were lots of anxious moments, but none like the weigh-in after an extended time at home. If you have seen the show then you can imagine what I am referring to, but for those who have not, I call it "Infamous Episode 9"...

After a two-week challenge at home, we all came back to California to a weigh-in. We had been told that each person who lost at least 5% of his or her body weight would be immune from elimination that week. If everyone met the goal, then no one would go home. Our time at home was tough, so no one was sure where he or she stood.

My team weighed first, and sure enough, I had not met our goal and was at risk of going home. The black team weighed in and only one person did not meet their goal. Because every other *member of the team had met the 5% goal and was immune from elimination, this meant that this contestant immediately went home - no vote, no discussion. This person was Chism, my son.*

Back at the beginning of this whole experience, on the night I packed to go out to LA, I suddenly had this thought that literally struck panic and fear into me. I said to Cathy, "What if somehow Chism gets sent home, and I am left there?" It had crossed my mind that I could be left alone on this crazy TV show, but other than that one moment when I was packing, I never gave it another thought. As I have said before, from the start I assumed that I would only be there for a few weeks. I would learn some stuff, get the kick-start I needed, and then let Chism get super healthy and be the TV star. His heading home first was not in the equation. However, this whole thing was not running on my plans.

This episode has been brought up to me by nearly every person I've met because it was so unexpected, so painful, and so powerful. I was crushed and left trying to figure out why I was suddenly there without him.

Essentially, I sort of lost it. I asked to take his place and threatened to leave, but two major things happened that changed my mood. The first was when I watched my son own his consequences and then challenge me to do the same. The rules stated clearly that he had to go, and I had to stay. As I listened to this young man call me out, I had no choice but to listen and humbly recognize the truth of his words.

The second was when Buddy calmly leaned over to me and said, "Chism needs to know that you support him." For a moment, I was thinking only of my hurt and myself and fully forgot that my son was up there hurting as he realized what had just happened. Buddy's words reminded me that I needed to show Chism I believed in him, and that with or without the show, he could succeed. I calmed myself and told Chism how proud I was, and that I knew he could do it. He was given an atypical sendoff with every single person hugging him and telling him goodbye. Tears were in abundance, not just from contestants but also from trainers, hosts, and the production crew. Nobody saw this coming.

When the emotion began to pass, the reality was still there. I was alone. I immediately began to question God and His purpose in all this. I had in my mind how things were supposed to go…and this was not it.

A Change of Plans

I learned quickly that day that God did not need my approval in order to do what He wanted to do. His plan was what mattered most. The problem was that I did not see His plan, or worse, I had tried to dictate His plan. I had this thing all planned out, and my plan seemed like a really good one. But now, He was getting my attention.

Every single day I spent time with God during this experience, praying, reading, praying more…so you'd think I would have let Him have full control. However, He was working on and in me when I did not realize it. As I prayed for Him to change me and make me the man I was supposed to be, He listened and was doing just that, but not the way I expected.

From day one, He started undressing me, taking everything away that hindered me from understanding this very basic principle: God matters. He matters. He exists, He loves us, He pursues us, and He cares for us. Knowing and experiencing this is part of the meaning of life. Everything is about Him, and everything should point us to Him. There is nothing that exists that is not used by Him to direct us to Him because He matters.

This is possibly the single most important statement in this book. **God matters**. He did not set this world in motion and then sit back to see what would happen next. He is involved and active in life. He desires for us to recognize and know Him. There is nothing else in this life that has greater significance than knowing this.

Distractions Are Everywhere

Our pursuit of things this life says are important all too often successfully pulls us away from the only thing that matters – knowing God through Jesus Christ. Unfortunately, this is especially true in the church. The church was never intended to be an exclusive club for its members to come and compare life. The church should exist as a place where people come together to share their bond in Christ, get trained and rejuvenated in their knowledge of Him, and then dismissed to go share their excitement with those who do not know Him yet. As the church this should be our message, God matters and you matter to Him. However, we seem to have gotten sidetracked to our purpose.

We all get overwhelmed and busy with life. One of the worst things about this is we slowly allow those things to impede our view of God. Unimportant things become important, priorities get out of whack, and life takes over. He knows this happens and continually uses things around us to draw us back. He does this with all of us because nothing is more important than knowing Him. He pursues all of us... even pastors on a reality TV show that should know better.

Alone on the Mountain

The next day was pretty rough. With motivation low and emotion high, the last thing I wanted to do was workout or do interviews. As we came downstairs we found there was another new twist. For the week, we would work with the opposing team's trainer. As if losing Chism was not enough, I did not even get the comfort of working with my trainer who knew me well and understood my level of pain and frustration.

We headed out to our "new" trainer for the week, and after a 4-hour workout, I found myself mentally, physically, emotionally, and spiritually spent. I leaned over a machine and just began to cry like never before. I was broken and just wanted it all to be over and done. I wanted everything else to go away and leave me alone, at least for a little while.

Thankfully, I was done with my stuff first and had time to myself. Uncharacteristically, I took off hiking on my own until I found myself at the top of a ridge all alone. After this experience, the absence from family, the lack of control, and feeling left alone, I absolutely unloaded on God. I let Him know clearly that I was unimpressed with His plan. I told Him this was not how I saw this coming together. I felt that what He was doing to me was unfair, unkind, and unnecessary - and I let Him know it.

What is amazing is that on that ridge I was not struck by lighting, rejected, cursed, or abandoned. On the contrary, I had the most overwhelming sense of His presence and peace. Never in my life had I experienced that kind of reassurance and grace. As I sat in the dirt, literally crying in desperation, my Savior showed up to let me know I was not alone.

*I realized everything up to that point had been leading towards this moment. He had been methodically undressing me from anything and everything that was keeping me from seeing that **He mattered most**. It was not God being mean, it was Him being persistent. The message He was trying to say to me was more important than anything else. Until that moment, I had* *missed it. I still remember walking down that mountain feeling like a completely different person. My resolve had changed, and I felt determined to continue this journey listening more intently to what He was showing me.*

It is interesting that after my time on the mountain, everyone said I was different. Literally, being on that mountain changed me, and I came down with a new vision and hope for what was ahead. I've read the story of Moses many times, but not until this day did I really get what his time on the mountain with God did to him.

At the time, I felt my time on the mountain had created in me a permanent life change, but after coming home I realized that letting go and trusting God was something I would continue to work on. (I'm human, and I will always need God.) I find that most things are out of my control and yet sometimes I convince myself just the opposite. Slowly I am realizing that ultimately I control nothing. God has it all covered, and my life only makes sense when I acknowledge that He is what matters. All I have to do is trust and look to Him.

I continue to learn that when you come to the very end of yourself and realize that God matters most, real life begins. He alone is the source of life and genuine life change. And yet, still. . .sometimes . . . I search.

The Search is Over

Recently, my daughter came rushing into our house looking for her phone. She went to her car, her room, the bathroom, the kitchen; she looked almost everywhere. Despite any attempts of mine to get her attention, she continued running around in a panic trying to solve her problem. Finally, she stood in front of me trying to remember where she was the last time she had it when she looked at me, and realized I had been holding it the whole time.

The point is I had it the whole time, but she was so busy with her plans for finding it that she never stopped and asked for help. If she had, then she would have realized at the very beginning that I was holding the very thing she was looking for. She would have saved lots of time and frustration if she hadn't been so caught up in her own stress that she couldn't see the key to solving her problem was right in front of her.

You are likely looking for the thing that will lead you to real, lasting life-change. It may sound strange, when you stop looking for it and instead look to God, you'll find what you're looking for. He has what you are looking for, and all that matters is putting your focus on Him. It is not always easy to relinquish control, but it will lead us to what matters most: knowing God and His plan for you.

MAIN POINTS TO REMEMBER

- **God has a plan for your life.**

  We've all heard this statement at least once in our lives, but usually we are too busy making our own plans to worry about what He wants for us.

- **Distractions are everywhere.**

  We lead busy, overcommitted lives and distractions come at us from everywhere, including the church. Remember who the author of distraction is and learn to say no to your plans and the plans of others so you can say yes to what God has for you.

- **God matters most.**

  If you don't remember anything else from this entire book, remember this, **God Matters Most**. He alone is the source of real life-change you are seeking.

Questions for discussion or thought

1. Have you had a time where life didn't go the way you expected? Think through that situation. How did you handle it?

2. What are the things you value in life? Make a prioritized list of what really matters to you most.

3. Are you willing to give up the things the world says are important and trust that God has something better for you? Why or why not?

4. If God has a mountaintop experience ahead for you, what do you hope is the genuine life change waiting on the other side?

CHAPTER 9

People Matter

"This is my command: Love each other."

– Jesus

B y now, you get the idea of where this is going. God matters because He first pursued us. But the next step is for us to realize that people matter. God made people; God pursues people. He would not make or pursue something that does not matter. So if people matter to God, they must matter to us.

It would seem to the outsider that people in the church should understand and live this principle better than the rest of the world. I cannot, and will not, speak for everyone within the church, but I will be honest and say this did not describe me. People did not matter to me.

Projects to Tackle, Not People to Love

Understand what I am saying, and see my transparency...I loved my family, my friends, and those I worked with and ministered to in the church (fellow pastors, parents, teens, etc.), but people outside the church were "projects," not relationships. I worked with the homeless, I worked beside many people in foreign countries to improve conditions there, I taught truth of Scripture in some unfriendly places, but I was completely missing the point. My purpose was never to figure out what to do for people; my purpose WAS the people.

If anyone digs into the life and teachings of Jesus, they will see this truth everywhere. Jesus had the ability to change everything for the people. He healed, He taught, He fed, and He challenged those in charge. He could have led a social change campaign unparalleled to anything before or since. However, we continually see Him stopping along the way and connecting with people. He knew them and came to share life with them. His agenda was less about changing their circumstances and more about letting them see what matters...Him.

I missed this. I was a judgmental Christian. It was us against the unsaved world. I had fully forgotten the meaning behind Christ's statement in His prayer for all of us, *"I do not ask You to take them out of the world...As You sent Me into the world, I also have sent them into the world"* (John 17:15 & 18). We represent Him to this world. I was never meant to separate myself from the world, but instead to let Him use me to transform the world. And how does someone do that? One person at a time...

I have found one of the most common questions I get is, "Would you do it all again?" Typically, it does not take me long to reply, "Absolutely." But my answer does not really lie in the reasons you may expect.

Obviously, the health/life benefits have been beyond expectation. Living life in your 40's and feeling better and doing more than you ever did even in your 20's is surreal. I love the fact that I have found the real me. That is worth it all, but that is not why I would gladly do it again.

That reason has to do with a close friend of mine named Jeremy. Jeremy and I did not know one another before the whole reality thing began, but seeing as he was another contestant in the house, we got to know each other very well, very quickly.

I have to be honest, there really is nothing Jeremy would not say. He is extremely comfortable sharing his opinion, sometimes in colorful ways. As a 'church' person, at first I was not sure how to respond to Jeremy. He was and is absolutely hilarious, but sometimes I struggled with whether or not it was okay to laugh. However, through months of life together with Jeremy, God helped me look beyond my Christian prejudice and actually see the amazing young man Jeremy was (and is), an amazing young man whom God was madly pursuing.

Jeremy came to our 'BLurch' in the second week and was unbelievably honest. He let Buddy and I know beforehand that he was not interested in buying any of what we were selling. (He had even told his grandmother before she passed away that he did not believe all this God stuff. It broke her heart, but he felt it was better to be honest.) He liked and respected us, and since Chism was his best friend, he came every week...and slept. I'd worked with teenagers for years, and none of them had ever warned me in advance that they would fall asleep. Jeremy's honesty was refreshing!

I will tell you this: Jeremy is a man of his word. For the first couple of weeks that he came, Jeremy pulled up a bench, grabbed a pillow, and dozed off a little. But then something crazy happened. Suddenly, he was not falling asleep. He was listening. Every now and then, he asked a question. Something was piquing his interest.

A Crazy Turn of Events

Then crazy stuff happened. Buddy and I were on one team, and Jeremy and Chism were on the other team. Through some of the drama of the show, Jeremy got switched to our team and he found himself working with a new group, a new trainer, and separated from his good friend Chism.

Then it got worse. Chism was sent home, and we were the only three guys left on the show. Follow me here...two pastors and a guy who told us to our faces he didn't believe in God...

There's no telling how many miles the three of us walked/ hiked together. At that point, we were the only three guys with seven ladies in the house. It seemed that drama was always around, so getting out and away was a great stress reliever. We talked nonstop. Sometimes it was about life or game strategy, but sometimes it was about God and our relationship with Him. Sometimes Jeremy asked questions, sometimes he just listened and walked, but he was always with us.

Slowly the number of contestants began to dwindle; yet the three of us remained - always together and continually talking. Finally, our time at the ranch ended, and we all returned home to wait for the show's finale in a couple of months. I was down in Texas while Jeremy and Buddy returned to separate sides of Michigan.

Because People Really Do Matter

During our off time, a really interesting thing occurred. Joe, one of the contestants, got in touch with Buddy and asked if he would perform the wedding ceremony for he and his long-time girlfriend, Anita. Buddy was of course humbled and excited, but as is typical of Buddy, he took it a step further.

Buddy's church ended up hosting 12 of our season's contestants so we could be there for Joe and Anita's wedding. He had people prepare a healthy dinner for their reception. Chism did music for the ceremony, I was honored to pray for the couple, and the local paper even provided free photography of the day. Not only was it incredibly special for the couple, it gave us all an opportunity to reunite. One of the contestants who made it to the reunion was Jeremy.

The Sunday following the wedding, Buddy's church opened the door for me to preach. Most of the contestants made it and the wonderful people of the community overwhelmingly welcomed us. It was a full house and a very special day.

As I closed the service, Buddy came forward to invite people to take hold of life in Christ. He explained that Jesus' grace covered all and the gift of life was available to anyone who just received it. The offer was there for anyone, and the hope was that some would find life in Christ on that day.

Then Buddy did something fantastic. He said, "We want to do this like we would on the show." He then explained how every week we would get on that scale with millions of people watching. Our progress, or lack of it, was displayed before the world. Nothing was hidden; everyone could see how our level of commitment had been. In the same way, he invited anyone who wanted to know Christ to stand where they were while everyone watched.

Now if you know much about church culture, this is unheard of. It is an unwritten tradition that everyone should bow their heads and close their eyes so that the people responding to the gift of grace can "feel comfortable". Through my years in student ministry, I knew there would be a few wandering eyes, but for the most part people respected the request. Buddy's statement was going against decades of church history, but I figured I'd just let him go for it.

UNDRESSED

While everyone else was watching, I chose to bow my head and pray for those in the room to take advantage of this moment. As a speaker, there is nothing greater than the moment when you realize that God has spoken through you to reach into someone's life for Him. I simply prayed that people would listen to God's prompting.

Then it happened. Cathy was sitting behind me, and I heard her crying quietly and moving around. I realized there were people standing in response to Buddy's invitation, and my heart welled up with emotion. Then Chism, who was sitting next to me, poked me, and I looked up and saw he was teary eyed. He motioned behind us, and as I looked I could not help but become overwhelmed.

Standing behind us, letting everyone know that God's grace has impacted him and that he wanted to live for Christ, was Jeremy.

This young man, who was thrown into our lives through a crazy experience and forced to endure unreal obstacles and changes along the way, had decided that he wanted to know Jesus. In that single moment, everything I had endured made sense. One of the greatest statements I heard him say was related to the fact that he couldn't wait to see his grandmother again someday. He just knew it was going to be a wonderful surprise and a great reunion.

When people ask me if I would do it all over again, I do not even have to hesitate. By the power and grace of God, my good friend, Jeremy, came to hear about and receive true life. If that was the only thing that had been accomplished through this experience, then it was all worth it.

Before this adventure, I was not very good with people. Even though my job involved relating with various types of people, I was never really good at making connections.

However, life is different now. I realize that people matter to God, and therefore, they should matter, **really matter,** to me.

This truth has completely changed me. Whenever seriously overweight people stop me and openly share about their physical struggles, I have a choice to make. I can either be freaked out and walk away, or I can engage and encourage them…I choose the latter. For me, every person I meet is a person God loves, and my goal is to make sure they know that, because people matter.

MAIN POINTS TO REMEMBER

- **People Matter.**

  God pursues people because they matter to Him. If they matter to Him, they should matter to us. It really is that simple.

- **People Aren't Projects.**

  What we do "for" people is not what is important. People are important. Treating them like they are a project to tackle or a problem to solve is not the example Jesus gave to us.

- **People Have a Lot to Offer Us.**

  Learning to accept Jeremy for Jeremy was so important to building our relationship. Imagine if I had distanced myself from him because I thought he was too outspoken, his humor too inappropriate or he was too different from me? I learned so much from Jeremy about truly accepting and loving others.

Questions for discussion or thought

1. How much of your life is spent truly engaging in relationships with other people? Why?

2. For some of us connecting is hard. What is your struggle in developing relationships with people around you?

3. Many times we do not see the big picture and do not realize what God is really doing. Is this you? How would you like to see God potentially use you in the lives of others?

4. Who in your life needs hope and encouragement? What will you do to share that with them today?

CHAPTER 10

Unexpected Rewards

"It is indeed hard for the strong to be just to the weak, but acting justly always has its rewards."

– Eamon de Valera

This is a strange but largely true statement: most trainers have never been overweight. Does that seem odd to anyone else but me? These people who have such a passion for health and fitness, by and large, have always been healthy and fit, which brings me to an issue of concern: how can they truly help me if they've never been where I am?

One of the greatest joys of the experience I've had in losing 100 pounds has been the connection with people. Not because I am anything special, but simply because they know I understand. I've been where many of them are so we are connected somehow. At least for now, I have conquered a beast that many of them are still fighting (they do not realize that the fight never really ends, but maybe that is a topic for another book).

Been There, Done That, Got the T-Shirt
(No, I actually got a t-shirt.)

I fully appreciate the heart of those who want to see us all get healthy and help us understand there is a better life ahead when we are fit, but there is something about having been through it that speaks volumes.

People ask all the time, "What do you eat?" "How much do you exercise?" "What's been the hardest part?" "What's been the best part?" All of these are questions of hope and connection. They want to know there really is a way to freedom from someone who has been through it.

Look at how this amazing truth translates to the example we see in Jesus! When I have this conversation with people, it is the easiest transition in the world to let them see how Christ chose to become a man in order to connect with us in this same way. He has been there (in heaven), and here (on earth) as God and as man, and He shown us all there is a path if we follow Him.

Some of my favorite people that I have met through my experience are the ones behind the scenes. There were so many people who truly loved and cared for us that never made it in front of the camera. These young men and women were there with us day in and day out, making sure we were awake, helping us through the process, driving us around in vans from location to location, and just living this weird reality TV show life with us. Their friendship is one that still impacts me to this day.

It has been awesome to learn that other seasons also had "church" as we did. It seems that when people of faith are in awkward, stressful, and uncomfortable places, we all tend to lean on our relationship with God. Generally speaking, I do not think we see the influence this has on those around us. However, I got to see a glimpse of this through my time in BLurch (Biggest Loser Church).

One of the examples is of an amazing young woman who was a production assistant. She began hanging out during our times together on Sunday evening, and shared with me early on that she really loved seeing how our faith seemed to be part of all of our lives. She grew up with a great family, but God was not ever a factor for them. Family was important, and they loved and supported one another, but thinking about - much less knowing - God was pretty foreign.

At one point in our season, this young woman was driving a group of us to the airport for one of our many adventures. I have lived my whole life fighting motion sickness so as was typical, I sat up front to avoid getting sick in the stop-and-go LA traffic. As we talked, she said something I will never forget.

"It amazes me how your relationship with God is such a part of who you are. Someday when I get married, I hope I find a man of faith, because I would really like to have that in my life."

I was floored. Honestly, I felt like I was struggling to survive each day and did not know if my relationship with God was being seen at all, much less in a positive way. And yet, here was this young woman saying she could see that God was real in my life, and because of that she wanted Him to be in her life as well. Who would have ever thought in the midst of this craziness that God was using me to reach out to others?

Immediately I told her, "You do not have to wait to get married to have this in your life!" She asked some questions, and we continued to talk more. I do not think I had ever wanted traffic to go slower in my life. I asked her if she enjoyed reading and told her when I returned I wanted to bring her some books that she might enjoy. She was open, and shortly thereafter we arrived at the airport and parted ways.

Upon my return, I brought the books with me and was so excited to give them to her. As soon as I saw her, I joyfully gave her the stack of promised books. She was thankful, but also a little sad. She told me that she had taken a new job with another show and was there that day simply to say goodbye to all of us. She felt like she could not take the books, as she did not know how she could return them.

When I told her that they were a gift she got teary-eyed. "You really want to just give these to me? Why?" I explained that what was in them would answer lots of her questions, and giving away some books was the least I could do. She accepted them and we parted ways. I remember praying for her, hoping that God would continue what He had so clearly begun. But sometimes we don't get to see how things turn out with the people God places in our life.

A few months later at the show's finale, I was so excited to see her again. She came to see how we all had done and to say "hello". One of the first things out of her mouth was, "I've been reading the books..." She could not wait to let me know that she had been reading through them. I introduced her to my wife, Cathy, and the two of them really hit it off. In the middle of this after-party, at a hotel in LA the two of them sat down and began talking about the books.

She told my wife she had gone to church just to see what it was all about. Her exact words were, "I felt like a puppy looking into a window at a restaurant...I could see they had something incredible, but I did not quite know how to get to it..." What an incredible description from someone God was pursuing.

She continued to ask questions and even dismissed people who wanted to interrupt her conversation with Cathy. We went *different ways at the end of that evening, and Cathy and I knew God was chasing her. Somehow, some way, He had allowed us to be part of her story.*

We still keep in contact with her, and I pray for her often. God used this strange experience to show a wonderful young woman that He is real and wants to know her. As we were in the midst of being changed, God was also using us to change others.

As We Have Been Helped

2 Corinthians 1 speaks to this as well when it says, *"Blessed be the God and Father of our Lord Jesus Christ, the Father of mercies and God of all comfort, who comforts us in all our affliction so that we will be able to comfort those who are in any affliction with the comfort with which we ourselves are comforted by God." -* (V. 3 & 4) Once God has comforted (or helped) us with our struggles, we can then go to those who struggle and share the comfort we have received. We are the best vessels of this comfort because we are evidence of His strength through a common battle.

What this means to us today is this: by choosing to be healthy and fit, we put ourselves in a place where God is using us to help others (students, adults, fellow youth workers). The victory and comfort we've received is passed through us. We can be used because of God's work in our struggle.

This gives Paul's words new meaning where we read, *"Most gladly, therefore, I will rather boast about my weaknesses, so that the power of Christ may dwell in me." -* 2 Corinthians 12:9 Remember, the victory is greater than the challenge. Make the change you need to today so that you can comfort and encourage others tomorrow.

How I've regarded my health and fitness has not only

affected my life, but also the lives of so many around me. While I should not take the blame for other people's choices, I have to own my responsibility in this. If I truly believe that our bodies are unique and special creations of God, I should not only take care of my body, but I also must challenge others to take care of theirs. As their pastor, mentor, teacher, parent, coworker, (insert label here), we have to remember that we are an example.

One of the weirdest parts of my Biggest Loser experience was when we left the confines of the ranch and brought the show to our home. The line between "reality life" and real life is seriously blurred when the television cameras are in your living room. My family never got caught up in the hype of it all though. We just had fun. We loved having all these new people around us, and no matter what their role was, we wanted them to feel at home with us. This was another opportunity to connect with others, and each of our family members opened the doors and welcomed everyone in.

There was one time in particular when we wrapped up filming in our home. We were about to have some family time outside of the viewing world, and all the crew was packing up and heading out. They all were so gracious and expressed their support as they left that day.

However, one of the team members stayed behind. He purposely waited until the rest were out the door and then wanted to visit with Cathy and me. His words caught me off guard. He told us he had grown up in a Christian home, and even though he was far from those roots of faith, he could sense our relationship with Christ was a very real part of our lives. Our warmth had renewed something in him, and he told us he really wanted to come back to his faith. He shared that he felt unbelievably welcome in our home and with our family, and loved how we let them all in and made them feel a part.

He told us that our actions reminded him of what he had been taught about his own faith in relation to others, and he appreciated us living it out in real life. As he left, he thanked us multiple times for our example and for our entire family's hospitality.

Cathy and I were a little overwhelmed emotionally. We both realized even more that this whole thing was bigger than us. We were simply treating these people the way we thought was right and never imagined God would use it to stir this young man's faith. We use this as a reminder, even now, that we never really know how and where God will use us. This memory is still one of the rewards we hold onto today.

We have to remember that as we work on ourselves, we are also being used to work in the lives of others. You can do this for yourself and for them. Keep moving forward and get ready for the unexpected reward that comes from connecting with others in this life.

MAIN POINTS TO REMEMBER

- **Loving others brings unexpected rewards.**

  Living by grace, trusting God, and loving others unconditionally bring unexpected rewards. It's truly one of the best parts of living out your faith, realizing you're making a difference in someone else's life.

- **God uses us to show Himself to others.**

  As Christians, we tend to polish up our good Christian behavior in the presence of other Christians, and turn on our churchy attitudes when we are around those who don't yet know Him. It's so important to remember that God is using us 24/7 to show Himself to others. Being "real" means allowing God to shine through us in real ways, not polishing up what we think God should look like. Authenticity speaks truth.

- **The impact we make on others is usually accompanied by an impact they make on us.**

  Some of my greatest memories (and lessons) from my time on The Biggest Loser came from people that God allowed me to impact. While He was allowing me to have an impact on them, their impact on me was often far greater. I have learned to be myself, to slow down and take the time for others, and to embrace the people that God brings into my life, no matter how crazy the circumstances.

Questions for discussion or thought

1. Is it difficult for you to imagine actually living the life you desire to live? Why or why not?

2. If God uses our weaknesses for His good then we should not be afraid of them. What are your weaknesses? Take a minute to pray and let Him have them.

3. If God chose not to remove your weakness how would you feel?

4. Our struggles give us experiences that prepare us to help others with a similar struggle. Based on your area(s) of weakness, with God's help, whom could you help and encourage?

CHAPTER 11

Life Outside Ourselves

"True happiness...is not attained through self-gratification, but through fidelity to a worthy purpose."

– Helen Keller

Since 2005, my family has had the awesome privilege of going to the Dominican Republic. These trips are not vacations, rather they are opportunities for us to serve and help children in impoverished areas. I can honestly say it is one of the things I look forward to the most each year. My role has been to plan, prep, train, and oversee the trip with our group each year, and there is not one part of the process that I dread.

The organization we partner with is called VisionTrust (www.visiontrust.org), and their mission is to help orphaned and neglected children around the world live for God and love others. This is lived out in various ways; spiritually, physically, and educationally, and it has been amazing to watch children's lives changed every year through this great ministry.

Serving in this way was and is a fundamental part of my life, but in 2011, this trip impacted my life in a significant way.

The summer before we headed off on this unbelievable

journey we were off to the Dominican Republic (the DR) for another trip of connection and service. As the trip leader, I had prayed for and planned most every aspect of our week. However, this year was to be different.

I noticed I was more tired than normal during our week. It is typically filled with early mornings and late nights so I was ready for that, but this year felt different. I look back now and realize I was most definitely in the worst shape of my life. Taking four different medications and topping 300 pounds made "normal life" uncomfortable. It was exponentially more difficult in this environment.

Our week was filled with the teaching, construction, and overall just connecting with the beautiful culture of the Dominican Republic. The climate was hot and humid (like always) - more than I was even used to from living in Houston, Texas - but in the past it had never really mattered, because the chance to be with our friends made it all bearable.

Unfortunately, that year, on the last day of our work, I was done. Physically, I felt terrible and could not go any more. I ended up spending most of the day sitting in a chair under a tree watching everyone else finish our work. I still remember the feeling of discouragement I felt as I watched everyone else savor our final day. It was so difficult to miss out on this time that I had helped organize because I had not prepared myself well.

These people deeply mattered to me, and more importantly I knew they mattered to God. My purpose was to share this with them, but because of my choices, I fell short of my own expectations.

Created for More

Ephesians 2 tells us that we are God's workmanship, created

in Jesus to do good works, which He has prepared for us. What this means is that each of us has been created with a purpose. God made each of us with a specific job in mind; jobs that will help make Him known to this world; jobs that are unique to each individual. While some of our purposes may look similar, ultimately we each have something to do that no one but us is meant to do.

Now hear this clearly, this is not work that brings us approval or acceptance from God. As has already been stated, there is nothing you can do to make God love or accept you more. He already loves you with a perfect love, and His grace covers everything (meaning we cannot do anything to change how He sees us). So this job, our purpose, is done strictly out of our love for Him.

I do not know which is worse, the fact that so many people do not know they have this amazing assignment, or that there are those who do know but choose not to try and fulfill it. It's one thing to be unaware of this truth, but it's totally different to know and ignore or avoid it.

For me, I was a half-and-half sort of person. I knew I was created for good works, but was unable (physically) and unwilling (mentally) to pursue them fully. The problem is that God is not a fan of partial pursuers. Revelation 3 reminds us that God would rather us be hot or cold, not in the middle somewhere. He wants us all in for His purposes, and He is looking for those who are willing to walk this life with Him. In the same chapter of Revelation it says that He is standing at the door knocking, looking for those who will pursue Him and His purpose for them.

This is where many of us seem to miss out. John 10 tells us that Christ came so we may have a "full life". This does not mean our every wish will come true, but it does mean we will only live a life that truly means something if we live it in Him. Many are content to know God from a distance, so long as He does not interfere with their plans or goals. What they do not realize is that real life - true life - is only found when we grab hold of His purposes for us.

You, You, You

The truth is this: life is not all about you. You are designed to live life outside of yourself. Your goal should be to live for God and love others. Truthfully, there is not much room for our own selfish desires if we strive towards this purpose.

A couple of months after this personally disappointing trip, I found myself in the middle of an extremely visible life-change in front of America. I was bound and determined to not let "me" get in the way of what God's purposes were for my life again.

What was interesting was this was completely opposite of what I was being told on a daily basis on the show. It was normal to hear that our motivation needed to be ourselves, we were not getting healthy for our family or others; we were doing it for us. Regularly we were told that this was a time for us. "Focus on yourself, determine to create a better life for yourself"

Now I really do understand what they were trying to say. Many had gotten to where they were because serving others had become their excuse for being unhealthy, rather than their reason to be healthy. We had to get that excuse out of our mind and do what would make us better - they just left out an important part. I had to get better and healthier to be better used for others. In my current state, I was not being of good use to anyone. This was about changing that state.

Early on, even as I heard these statements that were intended to motivate us, I realized my time there could not just be about me. It had to be for a bigger reason. There was a life out there that I was missing and a calling from God that I was not fulfilling. He was going to use my time on the show to teach me both of those things.

Being on The Biggest Loser was a confirmation that my lifelong struggle with my health was going to be used in accomplishing a greater purpose. I just knew it.

This change had to come so I could be better at living and serving. My motivation was outside of myself. The thing that drove me was the desire to be better: a better husband, father, and servant for God. I realized that for every person on the ranch (and back home) to be successful, they had to find this for themselves, but I was to become the messenger. Someone had to start challenging and encouraging others to know that God has something great in store for them too; something that will push them to live a life greater than the one they were living on their own, for themselves. And that someone was me.

Rise Up

A great quote by Stasi Eldredge speaks volumes to where my mind was, "Much of what He (God) allows in your life is not for you to simply accept, but to get you to rise up!" The things I had experienced in life were there to motivate me to let God move me above them. Everything works for a purpose, a goal, and an overall direction that is divinely created. We all have different roles to play in this journey, but these roles directly influence and affect others.

I have always had purpose, but I guess in some way I just thought I was supposed to float along and figure it out. I see now that this was never God's intent. We are to live a life above and beyond who we are, but we cannot know how to do this outside of a relationship with Him. We were made to know Him and share life with others so they can know Him as well. A life lived outside of yourself is a life lived within the purposes of God.

One thing that many people may not realize is that most of the people who come off of the show share a heart to give back to others. Many of us realize that there are countless thousands of people who want the opportunity that we had, and so many of us come back ready to help in any way we can. It is not uncommon to see former contestants working in gyms, motivating and encouraging others through speaking, and promoting national causes such as The American Heart Association, Breast Cancer Awareness, The Tears Foundation, and many more. Something about this experience either enhances or creates a desire to help others.

After my time with the show had ended, I found myself with the same desire. Because of my deep connection and love for the work of VisionTrust, through my trips to the Dominican Republic, I was able to approach my friend and President of the organization about how this platform might be used to further their vision.

We talked about creating some videos for me to use as well as for promotion on VisionTrust's end, but there was something there that was not quite enough. God had something else He was doing. One more thing He wanted to change in me.

During some of our discussions it became clear that as VisionTrust grew, there were staff needs they needed to fill. As we talked, I got excited as I realized that God was bringing me alongside this organization, not just to be a spokesperson, but also as an employee. After prayer and more discussions, there was no doubt that our family was being called to serve with

VisionTrust full-time. So, after 17 years serving in churches in the youth ministry world, I switched gears with life and began another new journey.

How We Fit in His Story

A couple of things are fascinating to me as I look at how this all came together. First of all, before being taken through my crazy experience on the show, I honestly do not think I would have been willing to change everything. God had to bring me through this, undress me from the things that would hinder His work, and then clothe and equip me with a heart, mind, and body that was ready to head out into something brand new.

The other part of this story is that He was calling me to do something I already loved. I have been really open with people by saying that my favorite part of student ministry had become planning, prepping, and leading our trip with VisionTrust each year. God was bringing me to a new role that would require some more life changes, but it was easier because of the passion and love He had been creating in me for years before. God's desire was to lead me through this change so that He could ultimately enhance His work by feeding the desire of my heart.

Psalm tells us to *"delight yourself in the Lord and He will give you the desires of your heart..."* I have found this overwhelmingly true. Be careful and notice what this really says. God is not Santa Claus, who is waiting to give you everything you ask for. Instead, as we focus on Him and truly seek His plan for us, He then creates desires in us that line up with His plan. As God took things off of me and removed things from me, I began to simplify my life and really look to Him as never before. When this happened, His plan began to unfold, and He fed my desires because I was delighting in Him.

This is not just something random that happened to me though! This is true for everyone. As each of us gives our focus and attention to Him, His plan is then made real in us. When we decide this life is not just about us, and we chose to live outside of ourselves, He not only begins revealing the "big picture," He also shows us how we fit into it.

Choose today to live your life outside of yourself. You have no idea the adventure that is awaiting you.

You too can make a difference outside of yourself. Take time today to check out VisionTrust's website (www. visiontrust.org) to see how you can help an orphaned or neglected child around the world. There is also a lot of information about how you can join me on a life-changing trip to serve the needs of others.

MAIN POINTS TO REMEMBER

- **We were made for a purpose.**

  God has equipped each of us with unique and special gifts that He wants us to use for His glory. The reason we search for "our purpose" is that we intuitively know we were created to do something significant with our lives.

- **It's not about us.**

  Taking the focus off of ourselves opens us up to real and lasting change. A simple goal of life should be to live for God and what He calls us to do.

- **There's more to life just our needs.**

  Living for something beyond what benefits us is the key to living a life that makes a difference.

Questions for discussion or thought

1. How does it feel to hear, "life is not all about you"?

2. What in your life would change if you chose to be more intentional about living a life that does not focus on you?

3. We need relationships that feed us as well as ones that feed others. What connections do you have where you are simply giving, loving, and encouraging, with no expectation of anything in return?

CHAPTER 12

Nothing Else Matters

"Life is really simple, but we insist on making it complicated."

– Confucius

Inspiration is a word I hear a great deal now. "Mark, your story is so inspiring..." "Mark, you've inspired me to make changes in my life..." "Mark, you are such an inspiration..." Honestly, it still feels weird when someone says these things to me. I do not feel like an inspiration. I feel like a guy who still battles everyday to own this new person he has become (albeit a guy with a pretty unique life-changing experience).

It is a struggle; one that I think will always exist. I spent 43 years training to be the person I was, unfortunately that does not just go away because of a 6 month TV show experience.

However, here is what I do not struggle with. I now know, better than any other time in my life, that nothing else matters but this: God gave me the opportunity to be on The Biggest

Loser because He wanted to teach me that knowing Him and connecting with others is what life is all about.

There is Hope

Since the show ended, the opportunities have continued to come in. I have absolutely loved traveling around the United States to encourage others on their health journey. Meeting new people has become one of my new favorite things.

Recently, while speaking at a local college, I was watching the students come in to find their seats, when one of the students caught my attention. Inside my head, something told me, "She is the reason you are here today." She struggled to walk and had to grab a folding chair because the stadium-style seating was not an option. She sat in the very back of the room with a friend.

As we started, the host asked people in the back to move forward, and I saw her face drop. She was trying to hide, but her plan was failing. As she got up to move, I approached her and asked if I could help move the chair. She was incredibly friendly and sincerely appreciated the help, even though it moved her much closer than she had planned.

During my talk she shared with the group how she loved the show and had been quite a fan of Chism and me. She listened and responded to my questions without hesitation. It was clear she was truly engaged in this time we had together.

The end of the talk came, and we ran out of time for my typical Q & A session, but I invited anyone who wanted to talk to meet me afterwards. I knew she would be coming to visit. A few people wanted to ask questions, some wanted a picture, and others just wanted to say, "thanks for coming," but the whole time she stood there behind the others. She was waiting for everyone to leave before we talked.

Finally it was just the two of us, and immediately she was excited. She told me how much she loved the show, especially our season. She asked about Chism, and if I had contact with any of the other contestants. But suddenly, in an instant, her smile turned to tears. She said, "I am tired of hurting. I am tired of thinking about how I look. I want to change, but I just cannot. I do not know what to do or how to start." My heart hurt for her just as it has hurt for the many people I have met who are struggling.

I told her there was hope, and that it began today for her. We exchanged email addresses, and I let her know my wife and I were there to help. She just needed to let us know how. Her smile returned, and we parted ways until I would hear from her again.

This amazing young woman just needed to know there was hope. In that moment, she was all that mattered. If she touched my heart that much, then I cannot even imagine how God must feel about her. She did not need weight loss tips or exercise routines. She needed to know someone was there to encourage and believe in her. What I am learning is that there are many others like her out there. Help and hope is available, and it begins and ends with Christ. Sharing this truth is my job.

You Know What Is Actually Inspiring?

The great, all-knowing, all-powerful, ever-present creator of all things wants to connect with us, and then use us in unexpected ways. To know that this same Creator loves and cares for us is where inspiration is born. Everything that has come from this experience is a result of His initial pursuit of me.

1 John 4 says that, *"We love, because He first loved us."* If

my story is inspiring to others, it is only because Christ was inspiring me first. None of this has happened so that I can go inspire others with my story of change, it happened so that more people could hear that God loves them, and that's the only thing that matters!

The reality television world is growing all the time. Average people are being thrown in to the spotlight more and more as producers come up with ways to highlight real people. Some may call it a "15 minutes of fame" moment and that is fine. Personally, I don't care how long God chooses to let me have this platform. All that matters to me is that I use every second of it sharing the truth that I know He has taught me. All that matters is living for Him and loving others. These truths are all that gives life true meaning. Outside of them, nothing else matters.

MAIN POINT TO REMEMBER

For those of you who have followed this story to this point, there is only one thing to walk away with.

- **Do what you need to do today to be the person you are meant to be tomorrow.** Live life knowing that outside of your relationship with God and your relationship with people. Nothing else matters.

UNDRESSED

Questions for discussion or thought

1. To get your focus on what matters most, you must first acknowledge where it is right now. What issues or circumstances in your life are taking your time an attention?

2. Often, God works on one thing at a time with us. What distraction do you think that He may want to work on removing first? What will come after that?

3. You have been equipped to connect with and help others. Where is your heart for others? How do you see yourself feeding into the lives of others?

4. Who around you needs encouragement, hope, comfort, or simply a friend?

I want to challenge you to set a reminder to pray everyday and look for ways to show the grace and love of God to the people you listed above. After all, when all is said and done, there is truly nothing else that matters.

CONCLUSION

"Now this is not the end. It is not even the beginning of the end. But it is, perhaps, the end of the beginning."

– Winston Churchill

Tomorrow Had Come

"This is it, this is my time. I am going to get healthy. I am going to make a change...tomorrow.

"Tomorrow morning I'll get up and begin this journey. It's my time, and this is it.

"Except, I am busy this weekend...that's a rough time to make a change like this, so right after the weekend. I am doing it, one more weekend of unhealthiness and then I'll start...

"But summer is coming pretty quick, and to do something new in the summer will be rough. I mean, with vacations and work trips I just do not see how I can be healthy...but I will try to get more exercise.

"So for the summer I just will not worry about how I eat, but I'll be more active, and then when the school year starts, it will not just be a new year for my students, it will be a new

*year for me. I can do this, I will do this, maybe...after summer...
hopefully..."*

But 43 summers came and went for me, 43 years of not
living a truly healthy life. 43 years of making excuses, 43 years
of losing some weight only to be followed by gaining lots of
weight, 43 years of not being all I could be for my family, for
my ministry, for my God.

Finally, there was no next year. My health/weight could
not wait for summer to come and go. I was tired of feeling
weak and miserable and knew there had to be a better way to
live life than this. Tomorrow had come.

You Know the Story

You know how my "tomorrow" turned out. My journey has
been pretty visible...okay it's been REALLY visible. My desire
to get healthy and fit landed me right in the public eye.

In many ways, though, my journey has only just begun,
and I am asking you all to join me. What the show captured
was only the start, only a taste of what Christ is doing with
me, and what He wants to do with you.

Maybe we can move forward together. It's time for everyone
to know the truth and live life differently. It's time to take off
all the things that are getting in the way of experiencing true
and abundant life.

A friend of mine shared this inspiration with me,
*"Sometimes what you are most afraid of is the very thing that
will set you free."* It can be scary to let God clear away the stuff,
but I am living proof that when He does it, life is never the
same.

Through this experience, I have been undressed of not only
excess body weight. The gracious hand of God has removed

expectations, mistrust, fear, and stress. What is even greater is what He chose to clothe me with in return: grace, focus, rewards, and passion for life. These are awaiting you as well.

When you undress and take off all the junk life puts on you, you will discover and begin to live this simple truth: God matters, people matter…and nothing else matters.

HOW TO KNOW GOD PERSONALLY

The Real Beginning of Your Journey

So much of what I have shared in this book hinges on a recognition that God exists and that He desires a relationship with you. If you are unsure as to whether you have that relationship, I have included this section to guide you to Him.

Copied from CRU: Campus Crusade for Christ. Learn more at http://www.cru.org.

What does it take to begin a relationship with God?

Devote yourself to unselfish religious deeds?

Become better people so that God will accept you?

You may be surprised that none of those things will work. But God has made it very clear in the Bible how we can know Him. The following principles will explain how you can personally begin a relationship with God, right now, through Jesus Christ...

Principle 1:

God loves you and offers a wonderful plan for your life.

God's Love: *"God so loved the world that He gave His one and only Son, that whoever believes in Him shall not perish, but have eternal life."* John 3:16

God's Plan: [Christ speaking] *"I came that they might have life, and might have it abundantly"* [that it might be full and meaningful]. John 10:10

Why is it that most people are not experiencing the abundant life? *Because...*

Principle 2:

All of us sin and our sin has separated us from God.

We Are Sinful : *"All have sinned and fall short of the glory of God."* Romans 3:23

We were created to have fellowship with God; but, because of our stubborn self-will, we chose to go our own independent way, and fellowship with God was broken. This self-will, characterized by an attitude of active rebellion or passive indifference, is evidence of what the Bible calls sin.

We Are Separated: *"The wages of sin is death"* [spiritual separation from God]. Romans 6:23

Scripture illustrates that God is holy and people are sinful. A great gulf separates us. The arrows illustrate that we are continually trying to reach God and the abundant life through our own efforts, such as a good life, philosophy, or religion -- but we inevitably fail.

The third law explains the only way to bridge this gulf...

Principle 3:

Jesus Christ is God's only provision for our sin. Through Him we can know and experience God's love and plan for our life.

> **He Died in Our Place:** *"God demonstrates His own love toward us, in that while we were yet sinners, Christ died for us."* Romans 5:8

> **He Rose From the Dead:** *"Christ died for our sins...He was buried...He was raised on the third day, according to the Scriptures...He appeared to Peter, then to the twelve. After that He appeared to more than five hundred..."* 1 Corinthians 15:3-8

> **He Is the Only Way to God:** *"Jesus said to him, 'I am the way, and the truth, and the life; no one comes to the Father, but through Me.'"* John 14:6

It is not enough just to know these three principles...

Principle 4:

We must individually receive Jesus Christ as Savior and Lord; then we can know and experience God's love and plan for our lives.

> **We Must Receive Christ:** *"As many as received Him, to*

them He gave the right to become children of God, even to those who believe in His name." John 1:12

We Receive Christ Through Faith: *"By grace you have been saved through faith; and that not of yourselves, it is the gift of God; not as a result of works, that no one should boast."* Ephesians 2:8-9

When We Receive Christ, We Experience a New Birth

We Receive Christ by Personal Invitation: [Christ speaking] *"Behold, I stand at the door and knock; if any one hears My voice and opens the door, I will come in to him."* Revelation 3:20

Receiving Christ involves turning to God from self (repentance) and trusting Christ to come into our lives to forgive our sins and to make us what He wants us to be. Just to agree intellectually that Jesus Christ is the Son of God and that He died on the cross for your sins is not enough. Nor is it enough to have an emotional experience. You receive Jesus Christ by faith, as an act of the will.

You can receive Christ right now by faith through prayer

Prayer is talking to God. God knows your heart and is not so concerned with your words as He is with the attitude of your heart. The following is a suggested prayer:

"Lord Jesus, I need You. Thank You for dying on the cross for my sins. I open the door of my life and receive You as

my Savior and Lord. Thank You for forgiving my sins and giving me eternal life. Take control of the throne of my life. Make me the kind of person You want me to be."

If this prayer expresses the desire of your heart, then you can pray this prayer right now and Christ will come into your life, as He promised. If you have any questions please contact me through any of the ways listed at the end of this book!

FOAQ'S – FUN AND OFTEN ASKED QUESTIONS

(Nope, you aren't the only one wondering these things!)

Do you still keep in touch with others from the show?

Absolutely. There are a few people who I don't hear from but most of the group still connects. Personally, I talk to Buddy and Kim with the most regularity. Buddy and I have even traveled some together to speak in different places across the United States. Many of the others still keep in touch via texting or Facebook.

Why did you leave the show?

That's probably a topic for another book...until then I'll tell you, but only if you do 100 burpees first.

What's a burpee?

A terrible, terrible exercise...it's worth Googling.

How is Chism?

He is doing pretty well. He has his own story that he continues telling in his own personal "Chism" way. He has developed a significant social media following and is regularly working on something to post online. He continues to work on his health and looks for ways to help others as well.

I would highly encourage you to check out his YouTube channel. Look up ChizCor and follow his journey as you enjoy his video blogs.

What do you do about excess skin?

Believe it or not this is one of the most common questions I get! Many people have an issue with extra skin once they lose lots of weight. We were encouraged to do a couple of things:

1. Wait about 6 months to a year. This ensures that you maintain weight loss and allows your body to do as much of the work as possible.

2. Wear compression shirts, shorts, or pants. This will hold the skin in and make it manageable especially when working out.

3. Look into skin removal surgery. This can be a great solution down the road, but it can be costly.

What do you do for exercise now?

A couple of things have really become a part of my lifestyle. I love to run and now regularly run 5k and 10k races. It is really something I love to do. I also workout at a boxing gym and have found that I love it! Biking and swimming are favorites for me as well, but if I have a choice you'll probably find me running.

FOAQ's – Fun and Often Asked Questions

Is Dolvett really THAT gorgeous?

Yes. Enough said…

Were the workouts really as hard as they looked?

Yes. I have never experienced anything like it. They became awesome and exciting but early on they were simply terrible. But, hey, they were worth it.

What was the hardest part of the experience?

This is a very common question and there is no hesitation in the answer; being removed from friends and family is the worst part. Learning to eat right gets easier and as you lose weight the workouts, in many ways, become fun. However, the day-to-day living with no idea about what is happening at home is sometimes unbearable. Homesickness is something that really never goes away.

Do you ever eat something you shouldn't?

Absolutely. I have a massive sweet tooth so sugar is a huge struggle for me. However, I've learned the keys are grace and balance. When I make a poor decision, I don't just give up until the next week. I let it go and move forward. Pretty soon the temptations get easier to resist. I still have my meals and days that are a struggle, but they are not the norm.

How can I connect with you?

I've had lots of opportunities to travel and speak to churches and schools across the country. If you are interested in having me come share with your group then connect via email – mark@sweatcor.com

Also, connect with Cathy and me and to find out how to move forward with your journey to a healthier life. Cathy and I, along with Chism and our teammate, Buddy Shuh, founded SweatCor to encourage you as you seek to live life the way it was meant to be. There are various ways to find us:

Website – www.sweatcor.com

Facebook – www.facebook.com/sweatcor

Twitter - @sweatcor or @marktcor

Also, don't miss our blog. We each love to share tips and encouragements multiple times each week. Head over to www.sweatcor.com/blog and subscribe today.

ABOUT THE AUTHOR

Mark has been married to Cathy for 24 years and they live just north of Houston. Life looks very different now for them and their three amazing children than it did before the show. They find themselves traveling to share what they have learned on this journey. They are continually sharing with churches, schools, and individuals to motivate and encourage.

Mark continues to work with VisionTrust International connecting people and churches with needy and orphaned children around the world. If you would like to learn more about how you can be a part of our work, check out www.visiontrust.org to see ways for you to help a child around the world! If you would like to know more about how you can join Mark on a trip to a VisionTrust project, check out the site for information or send an email!

CPSIA information can be obtained
at www.ICGtesting.com
Printed in the USA
FSOW01n0330301214
4224FS